"If you've grown tired of one-size-fits-all health advice that leaves you feeling disappointed, this book will feel like a breath of fresh air. Dr. Mindy Pelz will help you create a plan that's unique to your body and your goals. She combines groundbreaking research, powerful stories, and a clear guide to greater health."

— **Jessica Ortner**, *New York Times* best-selling author of *The Tapping Solution*

"Dr. Mindy is the Warren Buffet of fasting."

— **Jesse Itzler**, entrepreneur, *New York Times* best-selling author, endurance athlete, and an owner of the Atlanta Hawks

"I have never met someone who has more respect for the body and its innate intelligence to heal than Mindy. Her reverence for the body is met with an intense passion for helping people learn how to tap into it through the timing of fasting, eating, and detoxing. This way of living is the way of the future for all women if they want to truly thrive."

— **Danica Patrick**, entrepreneur and former race car driver

"*Fast Like a Girl* is an amazing book that is both inspiring and informative. It's a wealth of knowledge for any woman who wants to reclaim their health. It will leave you feeling motivated and ready to take on the world."

— **Megan Ramos**, *New York Times* best-selling author, co-founder and CEO of The Fasting Method

"Fasting is an incredible tool for longevity and healing. With *Fast Like a Girl*, women finally have a go-to manual designed specifically to their unique hormonal needs."

— **John Gray**, *New York Times* best-selling relationship author of *Men Are from Mars, Women Are from Venus*

"In her groundbreaking book, *Fast Like a Girl*, Dr. Mindy Pelz provides a much-needed manual on fasting specifically for women."

— **Elle Macpherson,** founder of WelleCo, humanitarian, supermodel, and actress

"At a time when all of us are looking for ways to improve our health and vitality, Dr. Mindy Pelz offers great advice. This book is about fasting, but also so much more. It's about our womanhood, our health, and our lives."

— **Marianne Williamson**, four-time *New York Times* best-selling author

"A much-needed fasting resource for women!"

— **Sara Gottfried, M.D.**, *New York Times* best-selling co-author of *The Hormone Cure*

"Fasting is such an incredible tool for our mental and physical health. Dr. Mindy is my go-to for fasting! She's teaching women like me how to tap into our innate intelligence while minding our hormones."
— **Alexandra Elle**, author of *After the Rain* and *How We Heal*

"It's possible to say good-bye to being tired and hungry all the time. *Fast Like a Girl* will teach you how long and when to fast so your hormones will support you instead of working against you. Welcome to getting your brain back and having to buy new, smaller pants!"
— **Dave Asprey**, author of four *New York Times* best-selling books, including *Fast This Way*

"Fasting is not a one-size-fits-all approach. Dr. Mindy Pelz is one of the leading experts in this area of fasting for women, and she truly understands how fasting is different for both men and women. If you're a woman and want to get the most out of fasting, then this is the book for you."
— **Drew Manning**, creator of the TV show *Fit2Fat2Fit* and *New York Times* best-selling author of *Fit2Fat2Fit*

"Fasting is such a powerful healing tool. In *Fast Like a Girl*, Dr. Mindy does an excellent job of helping women understand how they can use fasting to power up their hormones, as well as providing tips and strategies that are easy to follow and tailored specifically for women."
— **Josh Axe, DC, DNM, CNS**, founder of Ancient Nutrition and DrAxe.com, best-selling author of *Keto Diet*, *The Collagen Diet*, and *Ancient Remedies*

"Wow. Didn't think Dr. Pelz could achieve the same brilliance as she put forth in *The Menopause Reset*—but she did—going above and beyond. This should be required reading for any and every woman on the planet wanting to bring metabolic flexibility, vitality, and longevity to their life! Packed with good science, resources, and inspiration, this will be the gift that keeps on giving."
— **Nasha Winters, ND, FABNO**, best-selling co-author of *The Metabolic Approach to Cancer*

"Dr. Mindy has written the guide of all guides for women looking to improve their health by adding fasting into their life. Most importantly, she plans it all around their menstrual cycle. As a women's health and hormone doctor, I can't recommend this book and her step-by-step process enough!"
— **Carrie Jones, ND, FABNE, MPH**, head of medical education, Rupa Health

"When it comes to health, there's no cookie-cutter approach. This is especially true with fasting. In *Fast Like a Girl*, Dr. Mindy Pelz does a masterful job of outlining why women should practice fasting differently than men. Mindy provides practical steps backed up by science on how women at different stages of life can apply fasting strategies to balance hormones, reset their metabolism, and lose weight without having to deprive themselves. If you are wondering how to apply fasting for your unique hormonal needs, this is the book for you!"
— **Ben Azadi**, best-selling author of *Keto Flex*

"The nutrition and integrative health fields are increasingly recognizing the power of short- and long-term fasting in protocols for health and disease. However, too often the influence of cyclical hormonal patterns on metabolism and fasting physiology is overlooked. Dr. Pelz outlines here a strategy for optimizing the healthful impact of fasting in coordination with your hormonal cycles."

— **Zach Bush, M.D.**, physician (internal medicine, endocrinology, and hospice care)

"Dr. Mindy is such a wonderful women's health advocate empowering women, at all stages, to embrace their physiology and to stop apologizing for our own unique needs! Fasting is one of many tools that can help us thrive irrespective of our life stage!"

— **Cynthia Thurlow, NP**, author of *Intermittent Fasting Transformation*

"Wow! How refreshing! Dr. Mindy Pelz's book weaves patient stories with ancestral and nutritional research about the science of fasting and tied it together with clear steps for women to follow. Her words of truth delivered spot-on advice. I found myself saying, 'Oh, I'm stealing that.' A wonderful read!"

— **Annette Bosworth, M.D.**, founder of Dr. Boz, owner of Meaningful Medicine and author of *ANYWAY YOU CAN* and *ketoCONTINUUM*

"*Fast Like a Girl* is a must-have guide for resetting your hormones, aging beautifully, and looking and feeling fantastic. But even more importantly, following Dr. Mindy's guidance can have a profound impact on generations to come because fasting is the ultimate detox. Buy a copy for your daughters and granddaughters, teach them to Fast Like a Girl and help put an end to this epidemic of hormone imbalances, infertility, and ultimately the chronic illnesses in our children."

— **Donna Gates, M.Ed., ABAAHP**, international best-selling author and founder of *The Body Ecology Diet*

"Much like with exercise, fasting is an incredible, free healing tool that everyone can benefit from. What makes this book so unique is that women now have a fasting manual that will help customize food and fasting to match the needs of their hormones. In *Fast Like a Girl* Dr. Mindy not only makes the science of fasting easy to understand but lays out a whole new health paradigm for women and men to improve their lives in a myriad of ways."

— **Tony Horton**, best-selling author and creator of the popular P90X workout series

THE
OFFICIAL
Fast
Like a
Girl
JOURNAL

● ● ● ● ●

ALSO BY DR. MINDY PELZ

Fast Like a Girl: A Woman's Guide to Using the Healing Power of Fasting to Burn Fat, Boost Energy, and Balance Hormones*

The Menopause Reset: Get Rid of Your Symptoms and Feel Like Your Younger Self Again*

The Reset Factor: 45 Days to Transforming Your Health by Repairing Your Gut

The Reset Factor Kitchen: 101 Tasty Recipes to Eat Your Way to Wellness, Burn Belly Fat, and Maximize Your Energy

*Available from Hay House
Please visit:
Hay House USA: www.hayhouse.com®
Hay House Australia: www.hayhouse.com.au
Hay House UK: www.hayhouse.co.uk
Hay House India: www.hayhouse.co.in

THE
OFFICIAL

Fast
Like a
Girl
JOURNAL

● ● ● ● ●

A 60-DAY GUIDED JOURNEY TO HEALING,
SELF-TRUST, AND INNER
WISDOM THROUGH FASTING

DR. MINDY PELZ

HAY HOUSE LLC
Carlsbad, California · New York City
London · Sydney · New Delhi

Published in the United States by: Hay House LLC: www.hayhouse.com®
Published in Australia by: Hay House Australia Pty. Ltd.: www.hayhouse.com.au
Published in the United Kingdom by: Hay House UK, Ltd.: www.hayhouse.co.uk
Published in India by: Hay House Publishers India: www.hayhouse.co.in

Project editor: Melody Guy
Cover design: Julie Davidson • *Interior design:* Karla Schweer
Interior photos/Illustrations: Marisol Godinez

Cataloging-in-Publication Data is on file at the Library of Congress

Tradepaper ISBN: 978-1-4019-7787-0

10 9 8 7 6 5 4 3 2 1

1st edition April 2024

Printed in the United States of America

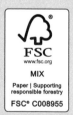

This product uses responsibly sourced papers and/or recycled materials. For more information, see www.hayhouse.com.

**To all the women who
are doing the work
to heal themselves.**

● ● ● ● ●

Contents

PART II:
Reflection Questions

PART III:
60 Days of Fast Tracking

PART IV:
Activity Pages

A LETTER FROM DR. MINDY

Dear Resetters,

Fasting offers a profound journey into yourself. If you are willing, it can be a beautiful partnership you enter into with your body. An agreement to trust, honor, and discover a wisdom that lives deep inside the trillions of cells that make up you. A wisdom that is always working in your favor, never against you. A wisdom from which the world may have disconnected you. Fasting can be your reunion moment. An opportunity to reconnect with the inner intelligence that is ready to heal you.

As you move through the pages of this book, keep in mind that you have been raised in a healthcare system that has taught you that health lives outside you, and that in order to be healthy you have to put something into you. All too often we lean in to the healing power of medications, supplements, or even food to move the needle forward on our health, leaving us unaware that it's our own innate cellular wisdom that is performing the healing magic. Although powerful, pills and food don't heal us. It's what our cells do with those external resources that heals us. Your cells are running your health show, and built within each cell is an intelligence that is more wise than all the doctors on the planet put together. Fasting gives you direct access to that wisdom. When you go into your fasted state, you are honoring this inner wisdom. Think of your fasting window as you telling your body "I trust you," "You know best what healing I need," and "I believe in you." At its core, fasting is reconnecting you to yourself.

While this journal will help you track the various aspects of your fast, it is so much more. I created this journal to deepen your connection to this inner wisdom. Keep in mind fasting can be a mirror. When in the fasted state, you often will see obstacles in your life that are holding you back, patterns of thought that no longer serve you, or maybe even situations in your life that need to change. This journal is designed to help bring forth an inner knowing that is ready to reveal itself to you. Without the noise of food, you will gain all kinds of insight. My prayer for you is not only will fasting help you create a body you love to live in, but that it reveals to you the steps you can take to live a life that is filled with joy, love, and peace. A life that you may have only dreamed of. Fasting can help make that life a reality.

From the bottom of my heart, know that I believe in you. I am cheering you on! I'm so excited to see what you discover about yourself as you move through the pages of this journal. You've got this!

Sending you a big hug,

Dr. Mindy

PART I

The Foundation

You Are Your Best Healer

Throughout my 25 years in practice, I have consistently seen that two of the biggest hurdles people come up against when trying to get well are time and money. Fasting takes care of both. I became so obsessed with this reemerging ancient health tool and the results I was witnessing that I decided to teach the science of fasting on my YouTube channel. I quickly discovered that many people, especially women, were also thirsty to learn how to fast effectively. Since then, I have been on the front lines witnessing a burgeoning health trend that has patients and doctors alike clamoring to learn more. Over the years, hundreds of thousands of healing stories have been shared on my channel. What has been clear is that people are falling in love with the results they experience when they fast.

Numerous studies have proven that outside of positive cellular changes, the most important part of improving your metabolic health is changing *when* you eat, not *what* you eat. Changing the time period in which we eat is more important than the actual quality of the food we eat. This is great news if we are to improve our metabolic health. Everyone can learn to take this fasting step. It doesn't take time or financial resources to fast. And you don't have to change your diet to better your metabolic outcomes. Something as simple as compressing your eating period will yield incredible results.

In this complex modern world, where food is available 24/7, is fasting the key healing tool we've forgotten? Change when you eat and you will undo the years of damage that poor living has done to your health. We've spent all these years debating which diet is best for humans, and it turns out, according to the science, that the best outcomes to our metabolic health happen not when we change what we eat but by the simple act of compressing our food intake into a smaller eating period of 8 to 10 hours. Think about this for a moment. Every diet you have ever been on has started with changing the foods you were eating or limiting the amount of calories you consumed, often putting you on a weight-loss roller coaster and perhaps even leading to great irritability and depression. Fasting changes the dieting game. That result you have been searching for through dieting can now be achieved through fasting.

But fasting's healing benefits go beyond the physical. So much insight stirs inside you when you fast. The wisdom that fasting brings to your life can clarify many aspects, like your relationship with food, the challenges you may be facing, and the creative ideas that have been building inside you that you haven't quite been able to access. Leaning into a fasting lifestyle offers you an

●●●

abundance of emotional, spiritual, and physical freedom. I created this journal to help you bring your truth to the surface while you fast.

Fasting invites you to receive the gift of spaciousness with your time and energy. You may even be surprised at how much time you spend shopping, preparing, and eating food. When you fast, you get that time back. For some fasters, the chatter in their minds while they fast can be a little distracting. This journal is here to help you productively channel those thoughts and gain deep insight and clarity.

One of the more beautiful aspects of fasting is that it deepens the most important relationship—the one you have with yourself. You get to know yourself in new ways. In these pages, I challenge you to document the unique aspects of yourself emerge as you build a fasting lifestyle.

This journey you are about to embark upon will be significantly enhanced by setting clear intentions for why you are fasting. A clear intention can be massively impactful if you are new to this lifestyle. Your brain will no doubt scream at you, "Go eat!" at some point on your fasting journey. The key is to remember that your body is in the process of healing and repairing. Having your intention written out beforehand is a powerful tool for staying the course when the hunger hits and the going gets tough.

Knowing and naming why you're doing this will shift a lot for you as you begin on this fasting-to-heal voyage. In my years of clinical experience, it has become extremely clear that when a person has a fierce "why," there is no stopping them. This journal will help you bring your own "why" to the surface so you have a meaningful target to focus on.

The inspirational thoughts that can come to you when you fast will help elevate your spirit and keep you focused on your fasting path. The brain can be a congested place. Navigating the chatter that goes on in your brain can be a daunting task.

Writing through the challenges and joys will open the door for deep self-inquiry. Be open to exploring your thoughts and self more deeply. As you write and reflect, you will discover some ideas you're ready to release— others may serve you well, and you will want to think deeper about them.

I hope this journal allows you to clarify the cloudy parts of your life. I hope it gives you an understanding of what you want to focus on and deep insight into problems you may struggle with.

As you work through these pages, remember you are worthy of self-reflection and inner peace. May your writing and reflection bring feelings of empowerment that you can accomplish anything you put your mind to and enable you to build a deeper connection to your heart's desire as you fast.

● ● ●

Fasting FAQ

WHAT IS A FAST?

You have two fuel systems that your cells get their energy from so you can function: sugar and fat. The first system, called the sugar-burner energy system, gets activated when you eat. Eating food raises your blood sugar. Your cells sense this influx of sugar in your blood and use that sugar, called glucose, as fuel for the thousands of functions they perform. When you stop eating, your blood sugar drops. This slow decline of glucose in your blood triggers your cells to switch over to the second energy system—called the ketogenic energy system, or what we lovingly call the fat-burner system. Very much like a hybrid car that switches from gas to electric for fuel, this switchover is when the fasting benefits begin. Although everyone will make this switch differently, research shows that it takes about eight hours after your last meal for your body to shift to its fat-burning system.

If you have never gone longer than eight hours without food, there is a likelihood that you may have never experienced the healing benefits of your fat-burner energy system. One of the most comprehensive analyses ever done on the science of fasting was published in *The New England Journal of Medicine* in December 2019. The authors reviewed more than 85 studies and declared that intermittent fasting should be used as the first line of treatment for obesity, diabetes, cardiovascular disease, neurodegenerative brain conditions, and cancer. It also stated that intermittent fasting has anti-aging effects and can help with pre- and post-surgery healing. This meta-analysis highlighted several key cellular healing responses that happen when we periodically flip our metabolic switch and move into our fat-burning system. These cellular healing benefits include:

- Increased ketones
- Increased mitochondrial stress resistance
- Increased antioxidant defenses
- Increased autophagy
- Increased DNA repair
- Decreased glycogen
- Decreased insulin
- Decreased mTOR
- Decreased protein synthesis

DO WOMEN NEED TO FAST DIFFERENTLY THAN MEN?

While the scientific evidence is clear that fasting heals, there still exists one huge blind spot: a one-size-fits-all approach to fasting doesn't work, especially for women. Women are highly influenced by the monthly and menopausal swings of hormones. The intricacies of our sex hormones—estrogen, progesterone, and testosterone—require that we pay closer attention to spikes in cortisol and insulin that can happen with an increase in stress, exercise, food, and, yes, even fasting. When we use fasting to flip our metabolic switch, we need to do it in sync with our hormones. Although men are hormonally driven as well, their hormones are not as sensitive to these spikes. For a woman to realize the full health benefits of fasting, she needs to know when and how to flip her metabolic switch in accordance with her hormonal cycles.

HOW LONG SHOULD SOMEONE FAST?

Intermittent fasting is typically thought of as going 13 to 15 hours without food. Yet many follow the research that's been done on 16:8 fasting—16 hours of fasting alternating with 8 hours of eating. Meanwhile, one of the most famous fasting studies revealed that a three-day fast can kill precancerous cells and reboot your whole immune system. As these scientific articles become more mainstream, and fasting becomes more popular, a lot of opinions are being tossed around on how long a person should fast. This makes it incredibly confusing for many to determine how long they should fast, if they should fast every day, and whether they are even fasting correctly. As you learn to thrive in a fasted state, it's tempting to go longer. But is longer better? Often there are no clear answers.

FASTING BENEFITS TIMELINE

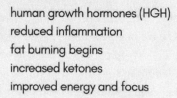 **INTERMITTENT FASTING**

13-16 HOURS

human growth hormones (HGH)
reduced inflammation
fat burning begins
increased ketones
improved energy and focus

AUTOPHAGY FASTING

17 HOURS

cellular detoxification
cellular repair
improved immune function
cancer prevention

GUT-RESET FAST

24 HOURS

intestinal stem cell regeneration
GABA production
brain healing
autoimmune healing

FAT-BURNER FAST

36 HOURS

reduced glucose stores
reduced insulin stores
increased fat burning
detoxification
anti-aging

 DOPAMINE-RESET FAST

48 HOURS

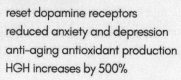

reset dopamine receptors
reduced anxiety and depression
anti-aging antioxidant production
HGH increases by 500%

IMMUNE-RESET FAST

72 HOURS

peak autophagy
immune stem cells
musculoskeletal stem cells
chronic conditions
accelerated healing

The Major Healing Responses Your Body Triggers While You Are Fasting

INCREASES KETONES

Ketones are an organic compound the liver makes when your blood sugar drops. They are an alternative fuel source for your cells when glucose is not readily available. A hallmark sign that your body is burning energy from fat is the presence of ketones.

For many, ketones are what they are chasing with their fasting lifestyle. You feel limitless when your body makes ketones. If you fear how you feel when you fast, know that once your cells have made the switch over to this fat-burning state and ketones are on the scene, your energy and mental clarity will increase. It's the opposite of any diet you have ever been on. When you train your body to make ketones, fasting will not only get easier but more healing will occur with time.

INCREASES AUTOPHAGY

Autophagy is a form of detox that has the ability to clean up our cells. Over time our cells accumulate a variety of damaged organelles, proteins, oxidized particles, and harmful pathogens. This accumulation causes our cells to become dysfunctional. When in a state of autophagy, our brilliant cells will detox these malfunctioning parts out of the cell, thus revitalizing them. This cellular reboot is a large reason why so many fasters feel younger and more vibrant the more times they dip into an autophagy state. Food will typically pull you out of autophagy, while longer fasts put you back into this healing state.

DECREASES GLYCOGEN AND INSULIN STORES

If you've been eating a high-sugar diet for years, your body has had to store all of that extra sugar somewhere. It stores it in a form of sugar called glycogen. There are three key places your body puts this excess sugar: muscles, liver, and fat. Think of it like when you make a big shop at the grocery store and not all of the food you bought will fit in your refrigerator, so you store it in a freezer in your garage. This is what your body will do with excess glucose.

It stores it as glycogen in your fat. Once you run out of food in the kitchen, you reach for the extra food in the garage. That is what your body does when fasting. You force it to go find the excess sugar it's been storing for years and use that for fuel. The glycogen stores in your muscles are easy to get to through exercise, specifically high-intensity interval training and strength training. But how do you get to the liver and fat stores? This is where fasting really shines as it is one of the most effective ways to release glycogen stores in your liver and fat.

Excess glucose is not the only thing your cells release when you fast. Fasting also forces your body to release excess insulin, which spikes every time you eat. If you eat a high-sugar, high-carbohydrate meal, you will experience a large insulin spike. Do this several times a day for years and you end up flooding your cells with insulin, thus making them insulin resistant. Like it does with extra glucose, your body has to store this excess insulin somewhere, so it packs it away in your liver and fat. Once again, the more you put yourself into a fasted state, the more you force your body to go find those insulin stores and metabolize them for excretion.

INCREASES GROWTH HORMONE PRODUCTION

Our body's growth hormone is our fountain of youth and it performs three key functions. The first is that it helps you burn fat, especially around the midsection. The second fabulous process that growth hormone provides is muscle growth. Have you noticed that your muscle-building efforts in the gym yielded results more quickly when you were younger? I can't tell you how many women over 40 I have heard complain about the muscle loss that occurs with aging. Once again, the disappearance of growth hormone will accelerate the muscle loss you experience with age. Lastly, growth hormone supports healthy brain growth. When you were younger your brain needed it to help it learn new life skills. After 30 you have learned most of the skills necessary to perform daily life tasks, so this hormone isn't needed anymore.

If you want to burn more fat, increase your muscle size, and have the brainpower to learn a new skill, fasting comes to the rescue. Depending on the length of your fast, decreasing blood sugar levels stimulates your body to make growth hormone fivefold, giving you back that youthful feeling.

RESETS DOPAMINE PATHWAYS

Every time you eat something yummy, you are getting a dopamine hit. In fact, sometimes you get the dopamine rush just thinking about that food. When we eat all day long, we get dopamine hits left and right. This raises what we call your dopamine baseline. As this baseline gets raised, you need more dopamine-producing experiences to feel good. Just like you can become insulin resistant from too much insulin flooding your cells, you can become dopamine resistant from using food all day long to feel good. In fact, the research on dopamine and obesity shows that some obese individuals keep eating all day not because they are hungry but because they need more food to get a normal dopamine response. Obese individuals not only need more dopamine to feel the satisfaction of food, but as they age they have less dopamine receptor sites available to receive the dopamine.

The good news is that several studies show you can reset your dopamine pathways with different-length fasts. Not only does fasting stop the age-related decline of dopamine receptors that obese individuals experience, but several types of fasts can actually make your dopamine receptors more sensitive. In some cases, new dopamine receptor sites are formed, increasing your overall feelings of contentment.

REPAIRS THE IMMUNE SYSTEM

One of the most famous fasting researchers, Dr. Valter Longo, brought the three-day water fast to the world's attention. His notable study was done on patients going through chemotherapy; he wanted to see if fasting would help repair the decimated white blood cells that occur with a chemo treatment. On the third day of a water fast he saw something miraculous happen: old, worn-down white blood cells died off and a new, energized group formed. It was a reboot to the immune system that anyone going through chemotherapy needs. That happened because of the release of stem cells into the bloodstream at 72 hours of water fasting. Remember, the body gets stronger the more it fasts. It does this to energize your body so it can go find food. The stem cells that are released at 72 hours ensure your body is working at its best so that your chance of finding food is at its best. Specifically, the job of stem cells released at 72 hours is to identify the worn-down white blood cells and make new ones to replace them.

IMPROVES YOUR MICROBIOME

Did you know your body houses 10 times more bacteria than it does human cells? These microbes have a tremendous influence on how your human cells function. It is estimated that you have more than 4,000 different microbial species living in and on you, 90 percent of which live in your gut. They help pull vitamins and minerals out of your foods, make neurotransmitters like serotonin to keep you happy, break down estrogen so it's ready for excretion, and constantly scan your cells for inflammation that might need to be lowered. Trillions of bacteria are all hard at work supporting your cells so they can function at their best.

Weight loss, neurotransmitter production, breaking down estrogen—these are only a handful of jobs these microbes perform for you on a daily basis. Microbes have a hand in everything from how hungry you get to the foods you crave. The more microbial diversity you have, the lower your appetite will be.

Fasting brings back the health of these microbes. It does this in four ways: it improves microbial diversity, moves microbes away from the gut lining, improves the production of bacteria that change white fat into brown fat, and regenerates stem cells that will repair the gut lining. (Brown fat is the fat that keeps you warm. It is also an easier fat to burn for energy.) All four of these factors are key if you are looking to lose weight. We also have evidence that longer fasts, like a five-day water fast, can dramatically impact your gut bacteria, specifically the bacteria that influences blood pressure.

REDUCES THE RECCURRENCE OF CANCER

In 2016, *The Journal of the American Medical Association* released an observational study that looked at more than 2,000 women between the ages of 27 and 70 who had undergone conventional breast cancer treatment. After analyzing this large group of women for four years, researchers determined that when women fasted 13 hours or more, they had a 64 percent less chance of recurrence of breast cancer. This is largely because fasting created a significant decrease in hemoglobin A1C, an indicator of blood glucose levels, and C-reactive protein, an indicator of inflammation. Very few drugs can offer that kind of result. This is how miraculous the body can be when fasting.

A daily commitment to longer fasting not only helps women who have had breast cancer not get a recurrence but may also help women avoid getting a breast cancer diagnosis in the first place. New fasting studies are emerging daily, and studies like this one give us hope that we will see more scientific evidence that fasting is a go-to tool in the fight against many cancers.

Six Different-Length Fasts

Not all fasts are created equal. With that in mind let's break down six fasts, the research behind them, and when to use them for your own healing journey. The six different fasts are:

- Intermittent fasting: 12–16 hours
- Autophagy fasting: starts at 17 hours
- Gut-reset fast: 24 hours
- Fat-burner fast: 36 hours
- Dopamine-reset fast: 48 hours
- Immune-reset fast: more than 72 hours

INTERMITTENT FASTING (12–16 HOURS)

USE THIS FAST TO:

- LOSE WEIGHT
- DECREASE BRAIN FOG
- INCREASE ENERGY

This is the most popular style of fasting. Most people's definition of intermittent fasting is going anywhere from 12 to 16 hours without food. Think of intermittent fasting as your entry point into fasting. It is the easiest fast to fit into your life and will yield you the quickest results. Many people turn to intermittent fasting when they feel weight-loss resistant or they get fed up with yo-yo dieting. When done properly, intermittent fasting is a huge step forward in getting your body to go back to burning energy from fat instead of sugar.

If you are new to fasting, here's your first goal: eat your food in an 8- to 10-hour time period, leaving 14 to 16 hours for fasting. Start by pushing your breakfast back an hour. Do this for a week, then push your breakfast back for another hour, and keep extending your fasting window until you are comfortably fasting for 14 hours. Some people find that for weight loss it's better to

• • •

move their dinner up an hour instead of moving breakfast back. That works too; it's personal preference. Eating too late and then going straight to bed can impede weight loss. Either way, the goal is to train your body to adapt to a longer period without food, with your first major fasting ledge to grab on to being 14 hours.

AUTOPHAGY FASTING (17–72 HOURS)

USE THIS FAST TO:

- DETOX
- IMPROVE BRAIN FUNCTION AND COGNITION
- PREVENT A COLD
- BALANCE SEX HORMONES

If there is one cellular process that has drawn so many to fasting, it's autophagy. When your cells register dipping blood sugar while in a fasted state, this incredible repair process kicks in. Why do your cells do this? To make themselves more resilient. Without the influx of glucose coming in, your cells respond by making themselves stronger. Autophagy improves cellular resilience in three ways: detox, repair, and the removal of diseased cells. There is much debate about at what hour of fasting autophagy kicks in. I like to think of autophagy as a dimmer switch that slowly gets turned on around 17 hours and reaches its brightest peak at 72 hours.

If I had a favorite fast, the gut reset would be it. Here's why: it's easy, time efficient, and has a major impact on your microbiome. When you are in a fasted state for 24 hours or more, it's long enough to get a burst of stem cells released into your gut to repair its inner mucosal lining, which may have been damaged from years of chronic inflammation. This is the magic length of fasting to start seeing significant changes in your gut health. This fast is the first point at which your body will make stem cells, and those stem cells will find worn-out cells and bring them back to life. People pay large amounts of money to get stem cells injected into their joints, skin, and injured body parts in hopes of regenerating those areas. You can get a similar effect by fasting.

Ninety percent of your microbes live in your gut. Extending your fast to 24 hours invigorates these microbes that are critical to your immune system and will help make neurotransmitters that keep your brain happy, calm, and focused.

FAT-BURNER FAST (36+ HOURS)

USE THIS FAST TO:

· MINIMIZE WEIGHT-LOSS RESISTANCE

· RELEASE STORED SUGAR

· REDUCE CHOLESTEROL

No doubt fasting has taken the world by storm because of what an effective weight-loss tool it has been for so many. As exciting as the weight-loss benefits of fasting can be, there is a subset of people who fast every day, often eating only one meal, and the scale still won't budge. In an effort to help, I started leading some women whose bodies seemed resistant to weight loss through 36-hour fasts. It worked like magic! That length of time turned on a fat-burning switch they weren't able to get with shorter fasts.

DOPAMINE-RESET FAST (48+ HOURS)

USE THIS FAST TO:

· REBOOT DOPAMINE LEVELS

· LOWER ANXIETY LEVELS

This length of fast is what I consider a mental health boost. As mentioned previously, fasting can repair dopamine receptor sites, create new dopamine receptors, and improve your dopamine pathways. There is also scientific evidence that fasting longer than 24 hours makes your dopamine receptors more sensitive.

For the past several years I have been leading my online community through different-length fasts. I call it Fast Training Week, where as a community we practice fasting for different lengths of time. And every time, the 48-hour dopamine fast seems to improve people's mental health more than any other fast. The interesting part of this length of fast is that the fast itself doesn't bring mental clarity immediately; rather it's in the weeks that follow when your whole dopamine system is regenerated that you will feel the benefits. Often just one 48-hour fast will do this for you.

● ● ●

This fast is often referred to as the three-to-five-day water fast. The reason many go up to five days is because at 72 hours in a fasted state your body regenerates stem cells. Revitalized stem cells are able to find injured body parts and make them anew. After three days of fasting, new and improved stem cells can have a dramatic healing effect on aging cells. And you will keep making those stem cells until you eat again. Many people like to keep going with their fast, extending it to five-plus days to maximize stem cell production.

6 Different Styles of Fasting

1 13–15 Hours

Intermittent Fasting

50g protein
20g net carbs
60% of calories
from good fat

2 17 Hours

Autophagy Fasting

20g protein
50g net carbs
60% of calories
from good fat

3 24 Hours

Gut-Reset Fast

50g protein
50g net carbs
60% of calories
from good fat

4 36 Hours

Fat-Burner Fast

50g protein
50g net carbs
60% of calories
from good fat

5 48 Hours

Dopamine-Reset Fast

50g protein
50g net carbs
60% of calories
from good fat

6 72 Hours

Immune-Reset Fast

Phased Refeeding
Step 1: bone broth
Step 2: Probiotic Food
Step 3: Steamed Veggies
Step 4: Protein

How to Use This Journal

Although we think of fasting as a tool for better physical health, there is so much more it can teach us. In the absence of food, you will get deep insight into your relationship to food and the level of trust you have for your body, and possibly learn how to interpret the clues your body leaves you as it repairs itself. With that in mind, I strongly encourage you to look at this journal as your fasting copilot.

When I work with a patient, I like to see the trends of both blood sugar and ketone levels while in the fasted state, both of which you can record on the tracking pages. Although tracking your numbers is not a requirement to succeeding at your fasts, it does help you get a deeper understanding of what your body is doing while in the fasted state. Tracking your numbers can also be a guide to let you know how much stored sugar you have and if you are staying safe throughout your fast. In addition to blood sugar and ketones, you'll be tracking other metrics including sleep, energy, and emotional state.

It's normal for your mind to chatter at you often while fasting. Although some thoughts that flood in may feel negative, they have a message for you. The Reflection Questions laid out for you in this journal are meant to help you interpret those messages from a mental, emotional, spiritual, and physical perspective. After reading through the list of Reflection Questions, you'll find space on the tracking questions to answer them. The mind chatter can derail you from achieving your fasting goals. Answering the questions will keep you on track.

I like to look at knowledge as my fuel source while fasting. I encourage you to do the same. I have included several charts to fill you up with knowledge. They synthesize many foundational ideas of what it means to fast like a girl. Ideas include how to break a fast, what your blood sugar numbers mean, and what healing is occurring each hour you fast. Look at these charts as inspiring you to stay the course. Compliance will be easier when the mind understands why it is doing an activity. These charts will help you deepen your understanding of how you can use fasting to heal yourself.

Fasting also can give you the gift of time. It's truly amazing how much time goes into thinking about, shopping for, and preparing food. While you are fasting, you are given that time back. Let's use that time for healing. I have included some coloring and other activity pages that can be a fun way to calm the mind chatter, open up your creative channels, and soothe your overstimulated nervous system. Lean in to the coloring pages when you need a peaceful moment. You may be shocked at how relaxing coloring can be. And don't be afraid to color outside the lines! The activities on these pages also prompt you to learn more about yourself.

Lastly, please know that I am here walking alongside your fasting path with you. I have sprinkled quotes throughout the tracking section of the journal with my favorite thoughts about the miracles that can happen when you fast. When you feel low on inspiration, pick up this journal and know that my words are there to lift you up. I know the miracles that await you when you fast. When doubt floods your mind, lean on my certainty. I believe in you!

Cheers to an amazing fasting experience!

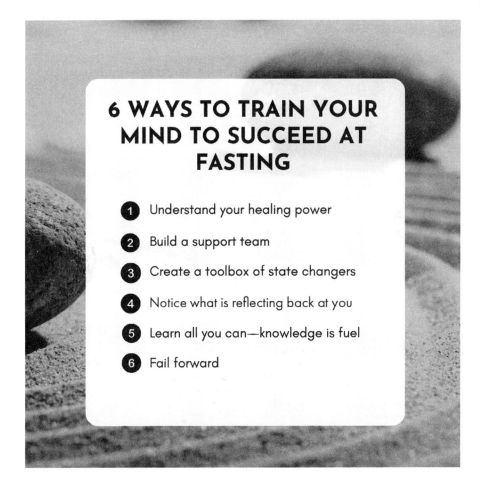

6 WAYS TO TRAIN YOUR MIND TO SUCCEED AT FASTING

1. Understand your healing power
2. Build a support team
3. Create a toolbox of state changers
4. Notice what is reflecting back at you
5. Learn all you can—knowledge is fuel
6. Fail forward

PART II

Reflection Questions

Mental

For many of us, food can become an unhealthy pacifier to our emotions. Often, we don't hear our feelings clearly when we are distracted by over- or undereating. Reflection during our fasts can help us find a balance and our personal truth when it comes to our relationship with food. When we go into a fasted state, we hear a voice that we don't hear when we're in a fed state. When we go into a fasted state, our inner voice emerges and tells us, *Here's how I use food. Here's the discomfort that I'm in. I'm not healing because I'm using food to quiet that voice.*

When we tune in, listen to our inner voice, and actually pay attention to what it's saying, we can often start to unpack what we are capable of. There's a language and a voice that comes to the surface that is hard to listen to when we eat. In this section, answer these questions honestly and openly without judgment.

1   Where in your life do you need clarity?

2   Where in your life are you lacking focus?

3   What thoughts show up when you're in a fasted state?

4   Are you kind to yourself during your fasts or hard on yourself?

5   What is no longer serving you? Dig deep.

6   What is fogging your brain right now and why?

7   How does fasting help you feel more grounded?

8   When you fast, what do you fill your mental space with? Is it helpful or hurtful?

9   Is the food you're eating clearing your mind or clouding it?

10   What do you want to discover about yourself when you fast?

11   How do you want to get to know yourself better in a fasted state?

12   Do you feel more connected to yourself when you fast?

13   How do you learn self-trust when you're not eating?

14   What thoughts feel hard when you're not distracted by food?

15   How has fasting helped you find self-control?

16 How do mental resilience and fasting go together for you?

17 What cycles are you breaking by fasting?

18 How does fasting strengthen your ability to choose yourself and your health?

19 When self-doubt emerges, how can you love yourself through it?

20 How do you use food to make yourself feel better and change your emotional state?

21 What scares you about not eating?

22 Where are you lacking self-trust when it comes to making food choices?

23 What messages around food were you taught from your upbringing?

24 What don't you trust about your body when it's in a fasted state?

25 How do you feel when symptoms of discomfort emerge during fasting?

26 What would it take to trust your body?

27 How do you not trust your body and why? Dig deep.

28 What is your greatest fear about fasting?

29 What would it take to love your body?

30 What thoughts keep coming up while you fast? Make a list.

31 What people are distracting you with their doubts about fasting?

32 What would it look like to live in a body that you love?

33 How would your relationships be different if you loved your body fully?

34 When you love your body, you are able to . . . (fill in the blank)

35 What information do you need to trust your body and your ability to fast?

36 How would life be different for you if you achieve your fasting goals?

37 How would your health improve if you kept your word to yourself?

38 What does it feel and look like to be proud of yourself? Make a list.

39 When do you give your healing power away to others and why?

40 What does it look like to come back home to yourself and reconnect with your truth?

41 What do you enjoy about your mind in the fasted state?

42 What comes easily when you fast?

43 Having more mental clarity offers you . . . (fill in the blank)

44 When you are not in pain, life looks and feels . . . (fill in the blank)

45 When you hit your fast goals, you feel . . . (make a list)

46 What does effortless health look like to you?

47 When you fast, you need . . . (make a list)

48 When you fast, you don't want . . . (make a list)

49 Who can you count on to support and uplift you when you're fasting?

50 When you're in control of your health, you feel connected to . . . (make a list)

Emotional

Honoring our body means paying close attention to how we are truly feeling, and the emotional aspect of your fasting journey is an invitation to rediscover just how powerful you are and what you're capable of. When you're fasting, you're healing yourself. You can't give the supplement or doctor the credit on this journey. You're the only one who can do this for you.

When you embark on a fasting journey, you must allow yourself to tune in to your feelings, thoughts, and emotions. Pay attention to what comes up. Don't turn away from the hunger pangs or the emotional distress you may face. All of this is information. Everything that comes to the surface offers you a moment to be honest with yourself and cultivate more self-trust. You will have to tell the truth to yourself because things will get hard. Use this section to unravel the challenges, lean in to self-compassion, and get to know yourself a little better. Honor the hard moments and be kind to yourself as you move through your fasts.

1   Why do you use food to self-soothe?

2   Where did you learn how to self-soothe with food?

3   What foods or drinks do you use to soothe yourself in unhealthy ways?

4   What feelings do you have about your body that you would like to change?

5   What in your life needs to change that is no longer in alignment with your health goals?

6   Who in your life is distracting you from your health goals?

7   What does it look like to feel grounded emotionally while you fast?

8   Where do you get joy from when you fast?

9   Where do you use food for social connection?

10   How can you make meaningful connections with people while you're fasting?

11   When do you distract yourself with food and why?

12   When do you find yourself mindlessly eating?

13   What triggers you to emotionally eat?

14   How do you use food for immediate gratification? Does that help or hurt you?

15   Does preparing food bring you joy? Why or why not?

16   Do you use food to procrastinate and escape from the hard things in your life?

17   Do you use food to numb yourself? Why?

18   What are you trying to numb when you're not in a fasted state?

19   What are you craving? (Food, relationships, work, love, creativity, emotionally, etc.?)

20   What does your emotional pain teach you?

21   How does joy serve you in and out of a fasted state?

22   Does your lack of health serve you in any way?

23   What emotional hurdles are in your way?

24   How can fasting create more self-reliance?

25   Who do you have to forgive to be healthy?

26   What emotional barriers are present in your life?

27   What are you hiding from?

28   What does being lovable look like?

29   What emotional benefits do you gain while fasting?

30   How does it benefit you to feel good in your body?

31   What feelings about yourself are you ready to release?

32   How will life look different when you let go and choose yourself?

33   What does emotional well-being look like in your life?

34   How does fasting support your emotional well-being?

35   What makes you most proud when you fast?

36   What do you learn about yourself when you're fasting?

37   How does your self-talk change when you are in a fasted state?

● ● ●

38 How can you use fasting to improve your confidence?

39 What does self-compassion look like for you?

40 Where do you need to forgive yourself?

41 How do you make emotional space to forgive yourself?

42 What tools do you need to start the self-forgiveness process?

43 What self-defeating patterns do you need to break?

44 What does fasting teach you about self-awareness?

45 How can you use fasting to heal emotionally?

46 What emotions are healing when you are in a fasted state?

47 What thought patterns are you untethering from while you fast?

48 How can you find more presence when you break your fast?

49 While you're fasting, what life decisions do you need to pay closer attention to?

50 What does fasting teach you about honesty?

Spiritual

To be able to hear yourself, your thoughts, or your connection to the Higher Power more clearly is sacred and beautiful. Fasting has been used for hundreds of years as a way to deepen spirituality, create emotional clarity, connect to God, and uncover answers that may feel far away. The Buddha sat under the bodhi tree, Jesus fasted for 40 days in the wilderness, and Islamists practice Ramadan. Even if you aren't religious, fasting can help you deepen your connection to yourself. There's something radical and transformative about that.

Some of us obsess about food in an unhealthy way by eating too little, by overeating to hide from our emotions, or by calorie counting and restricting to fit into toxic standards of beauty. Fasting in a way that is healthy and rooted in self-awareness can eliminate some of our core issues around food. It can bring us all closer to our truth and to ourselves. In this section, lean in to your spirituality and explore what that means for you and your life.

1   What spiritual insights do you gain while you're fasting?

2   How do you feel more connected to a Higher Power?

3   What spiritual teachings resonate with you in the fasted state?

4   How do you use fasting to prepare yourself for difficult situations?

5   How does fasting deepen your faith in yourself?

6   What are you most grateful for when you are fasting?

7   What do you want to purify in your life while fasting?

8   What are you the most connected to while fasting?

9   Who do you want to be more connected to while you are fasting?

10   What spiritual tools do you lean on when you're fasting?

11   How do you feel more connected with your breath and body while fasting?

12   Do your meditations/prayers deepen while you fast? If so, how?

13   Where can you surrender while fasting?

14   What do you hope to let go of when you're fasting?

15   How can you use fasting to discover your own spirituality?

● ● ●

16 Where in your life are you longing for a deeper spiritual connection?

17 Outside of food, what do you want to detach from while you fast?

18 How do you trust your intuitive guidance while fasting?

19 Where are you spiritually malnourished?

20 How can you use your spiritual beliefs as nourishment in a fasted state?

21 Where in your life do you need to cultivate more gratitude?

22 How does fasting help you be more grateful and present?

23 How are you grateful for your body while fasting?

24 Where do you need to be more empathetic with yourself and others?

25 Who in your life do you need to have more compassion for?

26 Where do you need to be more gentle with yourself?

27 What do you need to accept in your life?

28 What no longer supports your growth and healing?

29 Where do you feel spiritually blocked?

30 How do you want your relationship with a Higher Power to be? (Non-religious or religious)

31 What does spiritual love look like to you?

32 What rituals do you enjoy while fasting?

33 What brings you joy and fulfillment while fasting?

34 How does fasting deepen your spiritual connection?

35 How does fasting connect you to the spirituality of others?

36 What does fasting teach you about non-judgment?

37 What do you need to accept in the fasted state?

38 How does fasting help you accept and experience love?

39 How do fasting and forgiveness go hand in hand in your life?

40 What insights does fasting show you about forgiveness? (Situations, people, etc.)

41 What do you need to forgive yourself for in this season of your life?

42 How would your life be different if you forgave yourself and loved your body?

43 What does growth look like to you in and out of fasting?

44 How will you use failure to learn, change, and grow?

45 Where do you give yourself permission to fail without shame?

46 What does failure teach you, and what messages emerge?

47 What feelings of guilt and shame do you need to let go of to move forward?

48 What patterns of shame and guilt do you need to release to forgive yourself?

49 How would your life be different if you practiced more self-forgiveness?

50 What emotional baggage do you need to put down for your spiritual growth and healing?

Physical

We don't want to ignore the cues our bodies are showing us during a fast. Think of the body's symptoms as its own language. Its wisdom is speaking to you. It's your job to do your best to understand it. The physical part of fasting is a diagnostic mirror. If we listen close enough, we can lead ourselves toward rest or find the strength to push through. We have to listen and pay attention to what is in front of us. For example, if you notice that your energy tanks during your fast, you may have sparked your parasympathetic nervous system. What it's saying to you is, "Rest, slow down, and take a load off." When you leave your fasted state, pay attention to what emerges. Honor what your nervous system is telling you when you're fasting.

The physical manifestations we experience while fasting can be our greatest teacher, so that we can become our own greatest healer. Symptoms are our body's way of communicating. In this section, tune in to what's showing up physically in and out of your fasted state.

1   Do you feel safe in your body while fasting? If not, explain.

2   What does your body need to feel safe? Make a list.

3   What actions or changes are necessary to make your body feel safer during fasting?

4   Reflect on the messages you were taught about food growing up. What is coming to the surface for you?

5   How are the messages you learned about food impacting your fasting journey?

6   Do you feel like you have a good relationship with food now? If not, what do you want to change?

7   How do you decide when it's time to break your fast? (Things to think about: Are you bored? Are you hungry? Do you need a dopamine boost?)

8   Are there moments in your day when you unconsciously eat?

9   How do you want to be more mindful about what and how you eat?

10   Do you binge eat once you end your fast and open up your eating window? If so, why?

11   What would it look like to mindfully break your fast?

● ● ●

12 What's the purpose of food for you?

13 What part of your body are you trying to heal as it relates to fasting and breaking your fast?

14 How is pain showing up in your body when you fast?

15 What is your pain telling you? (Dive deep: Where is it manifesting in your body?)

16 How do you decide when to break a fast?

17 What brain changes are you noticing in your fasted state? (e.g., mood, focus, energy?)

18 What changes are you noticing in your digestive system when you fast? (e.g., bloating, constipation, cramping, diarrhea, etc.)

19 Are you having bowel movements while you fast?

20 What changes are you noticing in your joints while you are fasting?

21 If your body had a message for you, what would it be?

22 What part of your body needs more of your love?

23 When are you neglecting your body?

24 What body parts do you neglect the most?

25 What parts of yourself do you love? Make a list.

26 What do you want your body to look like a year from now?

27 What do you want your body to feel like?

28 How do you want to see yourself when you look in the mirror? Make a list.

29 What would a perfect day in your body look like?

30 What extra weight (emotionally and physically) are you carrying around?

31 How does the extra you are carrying serve you?

32 What is your fear around eating (overeating or undereating)?

33 What does your weight, regardless of the number on the scale, tell you about your self-worth?

● ● ●

34 How is weight protecting you from being seen?

35 What expectations of others are living in your body?

36 What is no longer yours to carry in your mind, body, and soul?

37 How does it serve you to stay in physical pain?

38 How will it liberate you to heal yourself?

39 What scares you about not being in pain?

40 How does your weight shelter you from being vulnerable?

41 How is poor health serving you? (e.g., do you get attention? Are you not held accountable?)

42 Do you believe that you are worthy of amazing health? Why or why not?

43 What does a healthy body feel like to you?

44 When you're hungry, what are you really hungry for?

45 What does optimal energy look like for you?

46 How does the number on the scale dictate your worth?

47 What clothes make you feel the most beautiful?

48 When you look in the mirror, what kind things can you say to yourself?

49 How does counting calories deprive you of self-trust?

50 What would it look like to love the body you're living in?

PART III

60 DAYS
of Fast
Tracking

FAST TRACKING

WHAT KIND OF FAST ARE YOU DOING?

IF YOUR FAST IS LONGER THAN ONE DAY, WHAT DAY OF YOUR FAST ARE YOU ON?

1 2 3 4 5

KETONE LEVEL
UPON WAKING

WHAT DAY ARE YOU ON IN YOUR MENSTRUAL CYCLE?

CIRCLE THE NUMBER THAT BEST DESCRIBES HOW YOU FELT AT THE END OF TODAY'S FAST

1 2 3 4 5

Angry Sad Neutral Happy Overjoyed

WHAT EXERCISE/ACTIVITY HAVE YOU DONE TODAY AND HOW DID YOU FEEL WHILE DOING IT?

WHAT WENT WELL DURING YOUR FAST TODAY?

IS THERE ANYTHING YOU'D DO DIFFERENTLY?

RECORD YOUR SUGAR VALUES

UPON WAKING

MIDDAY

BEFORE BED

HOW MANY HOURS DID YOU SLEEP?

CIRCLE THE NUMBER THAT BEST DESCRIBES THE QUALITY OF YOUR SLEEP

1 2 3 4 5

Very Low Low Neutral High Very High

CIRCLE THE NUMBER THAT BEST DESCRIBES YOUR ENERGY LEVEL

1 2 3 4 5

Very Low Low Neutral High Very High

BREAKING YOUR FAST

WHEN DO YOU PLAN TO BREAK YOUR FAST?

HOW DO YOU PLAN TO BREAK YOUR FAST?

HOW DID YOU FEEL AFTER YOU BROKE YOUR FAST?

REFLECTION QUESTIONS

Please refer to the Questions section and select an area (or two) that resonates with you. Then choose and answer a question from the area or areas that most align with your thoughts and experiences today.

AREA OF FOCUS	MENTAL	EMOTIONAL	SPIRITUAL	PHYSICAL

QUESTION

ANSWER

FAST TRACKING

WHAT KIND OF FAST ARE YOU DOING?

IF YOUR FAST IS LONGER THAN ONE DAY, WHAT DAY OF YOUR FAST ARE YOU ON?

(1)　(2)　(3)　(4)　(5)

KETONE LEVEL
UPON WAKING

WHAT DAY ARE YOU ON IN YOUR MENSTRUAL CYCLE?

CIRCLE THE NUMBER THAT BEST DESCRIBES HOW YOU FELT AT THE END OF TODAY'S FAST

(1)　(2)　(3)　(4)　(5)

Angry　Sad　Neutral　Happy　Overjoyed

WHAT EXERCISE/ACTIVITY HAVE YOU DONE TODAY AND HOW DID YOU FEEL WHILE DOING IT?

WHAT WENT WELL DURING YOUR FAST TODAY?

IS THERE ANYTHING YOU'D DO DIFFERENTLY?

RECORD YOUR SUGAR VALUES

UPON WAKING

MIDDAY

BEFORE BED

HOW MANY HOURS DID YOU SLEEP?　◯

CIRCLE THE NUMBER THAT BEST DESCRIBES THE QUALITY OF YOUR SLEEP

(1)　(2)　(3)　(4)　(5)

Very Low　Low　Neutral　High　Very High

CIRCLE THE NUMBER THAT BEST DESCRIBES YOUR ENERGY LEVEL

(1)　(2)　(3)　(4)　(5)

Very Low　Low　Neutral　High　Very High

BREAKING YOUR FAST
WHEN DO YOU PLAN TO BREAK YOUR FAST?

HOW DO YOU PLAN TO BREAK YOUR FAST?

HOW DID YOU FEEL AFTER YOU BROKE YOUR FAST?

● ● ●

REFLECTION QUESTIONS

Please refer to the Questions section and select an area (or two) that resonates with you. Then choose and answer a question from the area or areas that most align with your thoughts and experiences today.

AREA OF FOCUS	MENTAL	EMOTIONAL	SPIRITUAL	PHYSICAL

QUESTION

ANSWER

FAST TRACKING

WHAT KIND OF FAST ARE YOU DOING?

IF YOUR FAST IS LONGER THAN ONE DAY, WHAT DAY OF YOUR FAST ARE YOU ON?

1   2   3   4   5

KETONE LEVEL
UPON WAKING

WHAT DAY ARE YOU ON IN YOUR MENSTRUAL CYCLE?

CIRCLE THE NUMBER THAT BEST DESCRIBES HOW YOU FELT AT THE END OF TODAY'S FAST

1	2	3	4	5
Angry	Sad	Neutral	Happy	Overjoyed

WHAT EXERCISE/ACTIVITY HAVE YOU DONE TODAY AND HOW DID YOU FEEL WHILE DOING IT?

WHAT WENT WELL DURING YOUR FAST TODAY?

IS THERE ANYTHING YOU'D DO DIFFERENTLY?

RECORD YOUR SUGAR VALUES

UPON WAKING

MIDDAY

BEFORE BED

HOW MANY HOURS DID YOU SLEEP?

CIRCLE THE NUMBER THAT BEST DESCRIBES THE QUALITY OF YOUR SLEEP

1	2	3	4	5
Very Low	Low	Neutral	High	Very High

CIRCLE THE NUMBER THAT BEST DESCRIBES YOUR ENERGY LEVEL

1	2	3	4	5
Very Low	Low	Neutral	High	Very High

BREAKING YOUR FAST
WHEN DO YOU PLAN TO BREAK YOUR FAST?

HOW DO YOU PLAN TO BREAK YOUR FAST?

HOW DID YOU FEEL AFTER YOU BROKE YOUR FAST?

REFLECTION QUESTIONS

Please refer to the Questions section and select an area (or two) that resonates with you. Then choose and answer a question from the area or areas that most align with your thoughts and experiences today.

| AREA OF FOCUS | MENTAL | EMOTIONAL | SPIRITUAL | PHYSICAL |

QUESTION

ANSWER

FAST TRACKING

WHAT KIND OF FAST ARE YOU DOING?

IF YOUR FAST IS LONGER THAN ONE DAY, WHAT DAY OF YOUR FAST ARE YOU ON?

(1) (2) (3) (4) (5)

KETONE LEVEL
UPON WAKING

WHAT DAY ARE YOU ON IN YOUR MENSTRUAL CYCLE?

CIRCLE THE NUMBER THAT BEST DESCRIBES HOW YOU FELT AT THE END OF TODAY'S FAST

(1)	(2)	(3)	(4)	(5)
Angry	Sad	Neutral	Happy	Overjoyed

WHAT EXERCISE/ACTIVITY HAVE YOU DONE TODAY AND HOW DID YOU FEEL WHILE DOING IT?

WHAT WENT WELL DURING YOUR FAST TODAY?

IS THERE ANYTHING YOU'D DO DIFFERENTLY?

RECORD YOUR SUGAR VALUES

UPON WAKING

MIDDAY

BEFORE BED

HOW MANY HOURS DID YOU SLEEP?

CIRCLE THE NUMBER THAT BEST DESCRIBES THE QUALITY OF YOUR SLEEP

(1)	(2)	(3)	(4)	(5)
Very Low	Low	Neutral	High	Very High

CIRCLE THE NUMBER THAT BEST DESCRIBES YOUR ENERGY LEVEL

(1)	(2)	(3)	(4)	(5)
Very Low	Low	Neutral	High	Very High

BREAKING YOUR FAST
WHEN DO YOU PLAN TO BREAK YOUR FAST?

HOW DO YOU PLAN TO BREAK YOUR FAST?

HOW DID YOU FEEL AFTER YOU BROKE YOUR FAST?

● ● ●

REFLECTION QUESTIONS

Please refer to the Questions section and select an area (or two) that resonates with you. Then choose and answer a question from the area or areas that most align with your thoughts and experiences today.

AREA OF FOCUS	MENTAL	EMOTIONAL	SPIRITUAL	PHYSICAL

QUESTION

ANSWER

FAST TRACKING

WHAT KIND OF FAST ARE YOU DOING?

IF YOUR FAST IS LONGER THAN ONE DAY, WHAT DAY OF YOUR FAST ARE YOU ON?

1   2   3   4   5

KETONE LEVEL
UPON WAKING

WHAT DAY ARE YOU ON IN YOUR MENSTRUAL CYCLE?

CIRCLE THE NUMBER THAT BEST DESCRIBES HOW YOU FELT AT THE END OF TODAY'S FAST

1   2   3   4   5
Angry   Sad   Neutral   Happy   Overjoyed

WHAT EXERCISE/ACTIVITY HAVE YOU DONE TODAY AND HOW DID YOU FEEL WHILE DOING IT?

WHAT WENT WELL DURING YOUR FAST TODAY?

IS THERE ANYTHING YOU'D DO DIFFERENTLY?

RECORD YOUR SUGAR VALUES

UPON WAKING

MIDDAY

BEFORE BED

HOW MANY HOURS DID YOU SLEEP?

CIRCLE THE NUMBER THAT BEST DESCRIBES THE QUALITY OF YOUR SLEEP

1   2   3   4   5
Very Low   Low   Neutral   High   Very High

CIRCLE THE NUMBER THAT BEST DESCRIBES YOUR ENERGY LEVEL

1   2   3   4   5
Very Low   Low   Neutral   High   Very High

BREAKING YOUR FAST
WHEN DO YOU PLAN TO BREAK YOUR FAST?

HOW DO YOU PLAN TO BREAK YOUR FAST?

HOW DID YOU FEEL AFTER YOU BROKE YOUR FAST?

● ● ●

REFLECTION QUESTIONS

Please refer to the Questions section and select an area (or two) that resonates with you. Then choose and answer a question from the area or areas that most align with your thoughts and experiences today.

AREA OF FOCUS	MENTAL	EMOTIONAL	SPIRITUAL	PHYSICAL

QUESTION

ANSWER

FAST TRACKING

WHAT KIND OF FAST ARE YOU DOING?

IF YOUR FAST IS LONGER THAN ONE DAY, WHAT DAY OF YOUR FAST ARE YOU ON?

1   2   3   4   5

KETONE LEVEL
UPON WAKING

WHAT DAY ARE YOU ON IN YOUR MENSTRUAL CYCLE?

CIRCLE THE NUMBER THAT BEST DESCRIBES HOW YOU FELT AT THE END OF TODAY'S FAST

1   2   3   4   5

Angry   Sad   Neutral   Happy   Overjoyed

WHAT EXERCISE/ACTIVITY HAVE YOU DONE TODAY AND HOW DID YOU FEEL WHILE DOING IT?

WHAT WENT WELL DURING YOUR FAST TODAY?

IS THERE ANYTHING YOU'D DO DIFFERENTLY?

RECORD YOUR SUGAR VALUES

UPON WAKING

MIDDAY

BEFORE BED

HOW MANY HOURS DID YOU SLEEP?

CIRCLE THE NUMBER THAT BEST DESCRIBES THE QUALITY OF YOUR SLEEP

1   2   3   4   5

Very Low   Low   Neutral   High   Very High

CIRCLE THE NUMBER THAT BEST DESCRIBES YOUR ENERGY LEVEL

1   2   3   4   5

Very Low   Low   Neutral   High   Very High

BREAKING YOUR FAST

WHEN DO YOU PLAN TO BREAK YOUR FAST?

HOW DO YOU PLAN TO BREAK YOUR FAST?

HOW DID YOU FEEL AFTER YOU BROKE YOUR FAST?

● ● ●

REFLECTION QUESTIONS

Please refer to the Questions section and select an area (or two) that resonates with you. Then choose and answer a question from the area or areas that most align with your thoughts and experiences today.

| AREA OF FOCUS | MENTAL | EMOTIONAL | SPIRITUAL | PHYSICAL |

QUESTION

ANSWER

" —

You are
powerful
beyond
measure.

> As you fast, the longer you go ... the more healing switches get turned on.

FAST TRACKING

WHAT KIND OF FAST ARE YOU DOING?

IF YOUR FAST IS LONGER THAN ONE DAY, WHAT DAY OF YOUR FAST ARE YOU ON?

1   2   3   4   5

KETONE LEVEL
UPON WAKING

WHAT DAY ARE YOU ON IN YOUR MENSTRUAL CYCLE?

CIRCLE THE NUMBER THAT BEST DESCRIBES HOW YOU FELT AT THE END OF TODAY'S FAST

1	2	3	4	5
Angry	Sad	Neutral	Happy	Overjoyed

WHAT EXERCISE/ACTIVITY HAVE YOU DONE TODAY AND HOW DID YOU FEEL WHILE DOING IT?

WHAT WENT WELL DURING YOUR FAST TODAY?

IS THERE ANYTHING YOU'D DO DIFFERENTLY?

RECORD YOUR SUGAR VALUES

UPON WAKING

MIDDAY

BEFORE BED

HOW MANY HOURS DID YOU SLEEP?

CIRCLE THE NUMBER THAT BEST DESCRIBES THE QUALITY OF YOUR SLEEP

1	2	3	4	5
Very Low	Low	Neutral	High	Very High

CIRCLE THE NUMBER THAT BEST DESCRIBES YOUR ENERGY LEVEL

1	2	3	4	5
Very Low	Low	Neutral	High	Very High

BREAKING YOUR FAST
WHEN DO YOU PLAN TO BREAK YOUR FAST?

HOW DO YOU PLAN TO BREAK YOUR FAST?

HOW DID YOU FEEL AFTER YOU BROKE YOUR FAST?

REFLECTION QUESTIONS

Please refer to the Questions section and select an area (or two) that resonates with you. Then choose and answer a question from the area or areas that most align with your thoughts and experiences today.

AREA OF FOCUS	MENTAL	EMOTIONAL	SPIRITUAL	PHYSICAL

QUESTION

ANSWER

FAST TRACKING

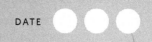

DATE

WHAT KIND OF FAST ARE YOU DOING?

IF YOUR FAST IS LONGER THAN ONE DAY, WHAT DAY OF YOUR FAST ARE YOU ON?

(1) (2) (3) (4) (5)

KETONE LEVEL
UPON WAKING

WHAT DAY ARE YOU ON IN YOUR MENSTRUAL CYCLE?

CIRCLE THE NUMBER THAT BEST DESCRIBES HOW YOU FELT AT THE END OF TODAY'S FAST

(1) (2) (3) (4) (5)

Angry   Sad   Neutral   Happy   Overjoyed

WHAT EXERCISE/ACTIVITY HAVE YOU DONE TODAY AND HOW DID YOU FEEL WHILE DOING IT?

WHAT WENT WELL DURING YOUR FAST TODAY?

IS THERE ANYTHING YOU'D DO DIFFERENTLY?

RECORD YOUR SUGAR VALUES

UPON WAKING

MIDDAY

BEFORE BED

HOW MANY HOURS DID YOU SLEEP?

CIRCLE THE NUMBER THAT BEST DESCRIBES THE QUALITY OF YOUR SLEEP

(1) (2) (3) (4) (5)

Very Low   Low   Neutral   High   Very High

CIRCLE THE NUMBER THAT BEST DESCRIBES YOUR ENERGY LEVEL

(1) (2) (3) (4) (5)

Very Low   Low   Neutral   High   Very High

BREAKING YOUR FAST
WHEN DO YOU PLAN TO BREAK YOUR FAST?

HOW DO YOU PLAN TO BREAK YOUR FAST?

HOW DID YOU FEEL AFTER YOU BROKE YOUR FAST?

• • •

REFLECTION QUESTIONS

Please refer to the Questions section and select an area (or two) that resonates with you. Then choose and answer a question from the area or areas that most align with your thoughts and experiences today.

AREA OF FOCUS	MENTAL	EMOTIONAL	SPIRITUAL	PHYSICAL

QUESTION

ANSWER

FAST TRACKING

WHAT KIND OF FAST ARE YOU DOING?

IF YOUR FAST IS LONGER THAN ONE DAY, WHAT DAY OF YOUR FAST ARE YOU ON?

1   2   3   4   5

KETONE LEVEL
UPON WAKING

WHAT DAY ARE YOU ON IN YOUR MENSTRUAL CYCLE?

CIRCLE THE NUMBER THAT BEST DESCRIBES HOW YOU FELT AT THE END OF TODAY'S FAST

1	2	3	4	5
Angry	Sad	Neutral	Happy	Overjoyed

WHAT EXERCISE/ACTIVITY HAVE YOU DONE TODAY AND HOW DID YOU FEEL WHILE DOING IT?

WHAT WENT WELL DURING YOUR FAST TODAY?

IS THERE ANYTHING YOU'D DO DIFFERENTLY?

RECORD YOUR SUGAR VALUES

UPON WAKING

MIDDAY

BEFORE BED

HOW MANY HOURS DID YOU SLEEP?

CIRCLE THE NUMBER THAT BEST DESCRIBES THE QUALITY OF YOUR SLEEP

1	2	3	4	5
Very Low	Low	Neutral	High	Very High

CIRCLE THE NUMBER THAT BEST DESCRIBES YOUR ENERGY LEVEL

1	2	3	4	5
Very Low	Low	Neutral	High	Very High

BREAKING YOUR FAST

WHEN DO YOU PLAN TO BREAK YOUR FAST?

HOW DO YOU PLAN TO BREAK YOUR FAST?

HOW DID YOU FEEL AFTER YOU BROKE YOUR FAST?

REFLECTION QUESTIONS

Please refer to the Questions section and select an area (or two) that resonates with you. Then choose and answer a question from the area or areas that most align with your thoughts and experiences today.

AREA OF FOCUS	MENTAL	EMOTIONAL	SPIRITUAL	PHYSICAL

QUESTION

ANSWER

FAST TRACKING

WHAT KIND OF FAST ARE YOU DOING?

IF YOUR FAST IS LONGER THAN ONE DAY, WHAT DAY OF YOUR FAST ARE YOU ON?

1   2   3   4   5

KETONE LEVEL
UPON WAKING

WHAT DAY ARE YOU ON IN YOUR MENSTRUAL CYCLE?

CIRCLE THE NUMBER THAT BEST DESCRIBES HOW YOU FELT AT THE END OF TODAY'S FAST

1   2   3   4   5
Angry   Sad   Neutral   Happy   Overjoyed

WHAT EXERCISE/ACTIVITY HAVE YOU DONE TODAY AND HOW DID YOU FEEL WHILE DOING IT?

WHAT WENT WELL DURING YOUR FAST TODAY?

IS THERE ANYTHING YOU'D DO DIFFERENTLY?

RECORD YOUR SUGAR VALUES

UPON WAKING

MIDDAY

BEFORE BED

HOW MANY HOURS DID YOU SLEEP?

CIRCLE THE NUMBER THAT BEST DESCRIBES THE QUALITY OF YOUR SLEEP

1   2   3   4   5
Very Low   Low   Neutral   High   Very High

CIRCLE THE NUMBER THAT BEST DESCRIBES YOUR ENERGY LEVEL

1   2   3   4   5
Very Low   Low   Neutral   High   Very High

BREAKING YOUR FAST
WHEN DO YOU PLAN TO BREAK YOUR FAST?

HOW DO YOU PLAN TO BREAK YOUR FAST?

HOW DID YOU FEEL AFTER YOU BROKE YOUR FAST?

● ● ●

REFLECTION QUESTIONS

Please refer to the Questions section and select an area (or two) that resonates with you. Then choose and answer a question from the area or areas that most align with your thoughts and experiences today.

| AREA OF FOCUS | MENTAL | EMOTIONAL | SPIRITUAL | PHYSICAL |

QUESTION

ANSWER

FAST TRACKING

WHAT KIND OF FAST ARE YOU DOING?

IF YOUR FAST IS LONGER THAN ONE DAY, WHAT DAY OF YOUR FAST ARE YOU ON?

1   2   3   4   5

KETONE LEVEL
UPON WAKING

WHAT DAY ARE YOU ON IN YOUR MENSTRUAL CYCLE?

CIRCLE THE NUMBER THAT BEST DESCRIBES HOW YOU FELT AT THE END OF TODAY'S FAST

1	2	3	4	5
Angry	Sad	Neutral	Happy	Overjoyed

WHAT EXERCISE/ACTIVITY HAVE YOU DONE TODAY AND HOW DID YOU FEEL WHILE DOING IT?

WHAT WENT WELL DURING YOUR FAST TODAY?

IS THERE ANYTHING YOU'D DO DIFFERENTLY?

RECORD YOUR SUGAR VALUES

UPON WAKING

MIDDAY

BEFORE BED

HOW MANY HOURS DID YOU SLEEP?

CIRCLE THE NUMBER THAT BEST DESCRIBES THE QUALITY OF YOUR SLEEP

1	2	3	4	5
Very Low	Low	Neutral	High	Very High

CIRCLE THE NUMBER THAT BEST DESCRIBES YOUR ENERGY LEVEL

1	2	3	4	5
Very Low	Low	Neutral	High	Very High

BREAKING YOUR FAST
WHEN DO YOU PLAN TO BREAK YOUR FAST?

HOW DO YOU PLAN TO BREAK YOUR FAST?

HOW DID YOU FEEL AFTER YOU BROKE YOUR FAST?

REFLECTION QUESTIONS

Please refer to the Questions section and select an area (or two) that resonates with you. Then choose and answer a question from the area or areas that most align with your thoughts and experiences today.

AREA OF FOCUS	MENTAL	EMOTIONAL	SPIRITUAL	PHYSICAL

QUESTION

ANSWER

FAST TRACKING

WHAT KIND OF FAST ARE YOU DOING?

IF YOUR FAST IS LONGER THAN ONE DAY, WHAT DAY OF YOUR FAST ARE YOU ON?

① ② ③ ④ ⑤

KETONE LEVEL
UPON WAKING

WHAT DAY ARE YOU ON IN YOUR MENSTRUAL CYCLE?

CIRCLE THE NUMBER THAT BEST DESCRIBES HOW YOU FELT AT THE END OF TODAY'S FAST

① ② ③ ④ ⑤
Angry Sad Neutral Happy Overjoyed

WHAT EXERCISE/ACTIVITY HAVE YOU DONE TODAY AND HOW DID YOU FEEL WHILE DOING IT?

WHAT WENT WELL DURING YOUR FAST TODAY?

IS THERE ANYTHING YOU'D DO DIFFERENTLY?

RECORD YOUR SUGAR VALUES

UPON WAKING

MIDDAY

BEFORE BED

HOW MANY HOURS DID YOU SLEEP?

CIRCLE THE NUMBER THAT BEST DESCRIBES THE QUALITY OF YOUR SLEEP

① ② ③ ④ ⑤
Very Low Low Neutral High Very High

CIRCLE THE NUMBER THAT BEST DESCRIBES YOUR ENERGY LEVEL

① ② ③ ④ ⑤
Very Low Low Neutral High Very High

BREAKING YOUR FAST
WHEN DO YOU PLAN TO BREAK YOUR FAST?

HOW DO YOU PLAN TO BREAK YOUR FAST?

HOW DID YOU FEEL AFTER YOU BROKE YOUR FAST?

REFLECTION QUESTIONS

Please refer to the Questions section and select an area (or two) that resonates with you. Then choose and answer a question from the area or areas that most align with your thoughts and experiences today.

AREA OF FOCUS	MENTAL	EMOTIONAL	SPIRITUAL	PHYSICAL

QUESTION

ANSWER

"

Your body is listening to everything your mind is saying.

"

People are so used
to being sick that
they have forgotten
what it feels like
to be healthy.

FAST TRACKING

WHAT KIND OF FAST ARE YOU DOING?

IF YOUR FAST IS LONGER THAN ONE DAY, WHAT DAY OF YOUR FAST ARE YOU ON?

1   2   3   4   5

KETONE LEVEL
UPON WAKING

WHAT DAY ARE YOU ON IN YOUR MENSTRUAL CYCLE?

CIRCLE THE NUMBER THAT BEST DESCRIBES HOW YOU FELT AT THE END OF TODAY'S FAST

1   2   3   4   5
Angry   Sad   Neutral   Happy   Overjoyed

WHAT EXERCISE/ACTIVITY HAVE YOU DONE TODAY AND HOW DID YOU FEEL WHILE DOING IT?

WHAT WENT WELL DURING YOUR FAST TODAY?

IS THERE ANYTHING YOU'D DO DIFFERENTLY?

RECORD YOUR SUGAR VALUES

UPON WAKING

MIDDAY

BEFORE BED

HOW MANY HOURS DID YOU SLEEP?

CIRCLE THE NUMBER THAT BEST DESCRIBES THE QUALITY OF YOUR SLEEP

1   2   3   4   5
Very Low   Low   Neutral   High   Very High

CIRCLE THE NUMBER THAT BEST DESCRIBES YOUR ENERGY LEVEL

1   2   3   4   5
Very Low   Low   Neutral   High   Very High

BREAKING YOUR FAST
WHEN DO YOU PLAN TO BREAK YOUR FAST?

HOW DO YOU PLAN TO BREAK YOUR FAST?

HOW DID YOU FEEL AFTER YOU BROKE YOUR FAST?

● ● ●

REFLECTION QUESTIONS

Please refer to the Questions section and select an area (or two) that resonates with you. Then choose and answer a question from the area or areas that most align with your thoughts and experiences today.

AREA OF FOCUS	MENTAL	EMOTIONAL	SPIRITUAL	PHYSICAL

QUESTION

ANSWER

FAST TRACKING

WHAT KIND OF FAST ARE YOU DOING?

IF YOUR FAST IS LONGER THAN ONE DAY, WHAT DAY OF YOUR FAST ARE YOU ON?

1   2   3   4   5

KETONE LEVEL
UPON WAKING

WHAT DAY ARE YOU ON IN YOUR MENSTRUAL CYCLE?

CIRCLE THE NUMBER THAT BEST DESCRIBES HOW YOU FELT AT THE END OF TODAY'S FAST

1	2	3	4	5
Angry	Sad	Neutral	Happy	Overjoyed

WHAT EXERCISE/ACTIVITY HAVE YOU DONE TODAY AND HOW DID YOU FEEL WHILE DOING IT?

WHAT WENT WELL DURING YOUR FAST TODAY?

IS THERE ANYTHING YOU'D DO DIFFERENTLY?

RECORD YOUR SUGAR VALUES

UPON WAKING

MIDDAY

BEFORE BED

HOW MANY HOURS DID YOU SLEEP?

CIRCLE THE NUMBER THAT BEST DESCRIBES THE QUALITY OF YOUR SLEEP

1	2	3	4	5
Very Low	Low	Neutral	High	Very High

CIRCLE THE NUMBER THAT BEST DESCRIBES YOUR ENERGY LEVEL

1	2	3	4	5
Very Low	Low	Neutral	High	Very High

BREAKING YOUR FAST
WHEN DO YOU PLAN TO BREAK YOUR FAST?

HOW DO YOU PLAN TO BREAK YOUR FAST?

HOW DID YOU FEEL AFTER YOU BROKE YOUR FAST?

REFLECTION QUESTIONS

Please refer to the Questions section and select an area (or two) that resonates with you. Then choose and answer a question from the area or areas that most align with your thoughts and experiences today.

AREA OF FOCUS	MENTAL	EMOTIONAL	SPIRITUAL	PHYSICAL

QUESTION

ANSWER

FAST TRACKING

WHAT KIND OF FAST ARE YOU DOING?

IF YOUR FAST IS LONGER THAN ONE DAY, WHAT DAY OF YOUR FAST ARE YOU ON?

(1) (2) (3) (4) (5)

KETONE LEVEL
UPON WAKING

WHAT DAY ARE YOU ON IN YOUR MENSTRUAL CYCLE?

CIRCLE THE NUMBER THAT BEST DESCRIBES HOW YOU FELT AT THE END OF TODAY'S FAST

(1) (2) (3) (4) (5)

Angry   Sad   Neutral   Happy   Overjoyed

WHAT EXERCISE/ACTIVITY HAVE YOU DONE TODAY AND HOW DID YOU FEEL WHILE DOING IT?

WHAT WENT WELL DURING YOUR FAST TODAY?

IS THERE ANYTHING YOU'D DO DIFFERENTLY?

RECORD YOUR SUGAR VALUES

UPON WAKING

MIDDAY

BEFORE BED

HOW MANY HOURS DID YOU SLEEP?

CIRCLE THE NUMBER THAT BEST DESCRIBES THE QUALITY OF YOUR SLEEP

(1) (2) (3) (4) (5)

Very Low   Low   Neutral   High   Very High

CIRCLE THE NUMBER THAT BEST DESCRIBES YOUR ENERGY LEVEL

(1) (2) (3) (4) (5)

Very Low   Low   Neutral   High   Very High

BREAKING YOUR FAST
WHEN DO YOU PLAN TO BREAK YOUR FAST?

HOW DO YOU PLAN TO BREAK YOUR FAST?

HOW DID YOU FEEL AFTER YOU BROKE YOUR FAST?

REFLECTION QUESTIONS

Please refer to the Questions section and select an area (or two) that resonates with you. Then choose and answer a question from the area or areas that most align with your thoughts and experiences today.

AREA OF FOCUS	MENTAL	EMOTIONAL	SPIRITUAL	PHYSICAL

QUESTION

ANSWER

FAST TRACKING

DATE ● ● ●

WHAT KIND OF FAST ARE YOU DOING?

IF YOUR FAST IS LONGER THAN ONE DAY, WHAT DAY OF YOUR FAST ARE YOU ON?

(1) (2) (3) (4) (5)

KETONE LEVEL
UPON WAKING

WHAT DAY ARE YOU ON IN YOUR MENSTRUAL CYCLE?

CIRCLE THE NUMBER THAT BEST DESCRIBES HOW YOU FELT AT THE END OF TODAY'S FAST

(1) (2) (3) (4) (5)

Angry Sad Neutral Happy Overjoyed

WHAT EXERCISE/ACTIVITY HAVE YOU DONE TODAY AND HOW DID YOU FEEL WHILE DOING IT?

WHAT WENT WELL DURING YOUR FAST TODAY?

IS THERE ANYTHING YOU'D DO DIFFERENTLY?

RECORD YOUR SUGAR VALUES

UPON WAKING

MIDDAY

BEFORE BED

HOW MANY HOURS DID YOU SLEEP?

CIRCLE THE NUMBER THAT BEST DESCRIBES THE QUALITY OF YOUR SLEEP

(1) (2) (3) (4) (5)

Very Low Low Neutral High Very High

CIRCLE THE NUMBER THAT BEST DESCRIBES YOUR ENERGY LEVEL

(1) (2) (3) (4) (5)

Very Low Low Neutral High Very High

BREAKING YOUR FAST
WHEN DO YOU PLAN TO BREAK YOUR FAST?

HOW DO YOU PLAN TO BREAK YOUR FAST?

HOW DID YOU FEEL AFTER YOU BROKE YOUR FAST?

● ● ●

REFLECTION QUESTIONS

Please refer to the Questions section and select an area (or two) that resonates with you. Then choose and answer a question from the area or areas that most align with your thoughts and experiences today.

AREA OF FOCUS	MENTAL	EMOTIONAL	SPIRITUAL	PHYSICAL

QUESTION

ANSWER

FAST TRACKING

WHAT KIND OF FAST ARE YOU DOING?

IF YOUR FAST IS LONGER THAN ONE DAY, WHAT DAY OF YOUR FAST ARE YOU ON?

1   2   3   4   5

KETONE LEVEL
UPON WAKING

WHAT DAY ARE YOU ON IN YOUR MENSTRUAL CYCLE?

CIRCLE THE NUMBER THAT BEST DESCRIBES HOW YOU FELT AT THE END OF TODAY'S FAST

1	2	3	4	5
Angry	Sad	Neutral	Happy	Overjoyed

WHAT EXERCISE/ACTIVITY HAVE YOU DONE TODAY AND HOW DID YOU FEEL WHILE DOING IT?

WHAT WENT WELL DURING YOUR FAST TODAY?

IS THERE ANYTHING YOU'D DO DIFFERENTLY?

RECORD YOUR SUGAR VALUES

UPON WAKING

MIDDAY

BEFORE BED

HOW MANY HOURS DID YOU SLEEP?

CIRCLE THE NUMBER THAT BEST DESCRIBES THE QUALITY OF YOUR SLEEP

1	2	3	4	5
Very Low	Low	Neutral	High	Very High

CIRCLE THE NUMBER THAT BEST DESCRIBES YOUR ENERGY LEVEL

1	2	3	4	5
Very Low	Low	Neutral	High	Very High

BREAKING YOUR FAST
WHEN DO YOU PLAN TO BREAK YOUR FAST?

HOW DO YOU PLAN TO BREAK YOUR FAST?

HOW DID YOU FEEL AFTER YOU BROKE YOUR FAST?

REFLECTION QUESTIONS

Please refer to the Questions section and select an area (or two) that resonates with you. Then choose and answer a question from the area or areas that most align with your thoughts and experiences today.

AREA OF FOCUS	MENTAL	EMOTIONAL	SPIRITUAL	PHYSICAL

QUESTION

ANSWER

DATE ● ● ●

WHAT KIND OF FAST ARE YOU DOING?

IF YOUR FAST IS LONGER THAN ONE DAY, WHAT DAY OF YOUR FAST ARE YOU ON?

1   2   3   4   5

KETONE LEVEL
UPON WAKING

WHAT DAY ARE YOU ON IN YOUR MENSTRUAL CYCLE?

CIRCLE THE NUMBER THAT BEST DESCRIBES HOW YOU FELT AT THE END OF TODAY'S FAST

1   2   3   4   5

Angry   Sad   Neutral   Happy   Overjoyed

WHAT EXERCISE/ACTIVITY HAVE YOU DONE TODAY AND HOW DID YOU FEEL WHILE DOING IT?

WHAT WENT WELL DURING YOUR FAST TODAY?

IS THERE ANYTHING YOU'D DO DIFFERENTLY?

RECORD YOUR SUGAR VALUES

UPON WAKING

MIDDAY

BEFORE BED

HOW MANY HOURS DID YOU SLEEP?

CIRCLE THE NUMBER THAT BEST DESCRIBES THE QUALITY OF YOUR SLEEP

1   2   3   4   5

Very Low   Low   Neutral   High   Very High

CIRCLE THE NUMBER THAT BEST DESCRIBES YOUR ENERGY LEVEL

1   2   3   4   5

Very Low   Low   Neutral   High   Very High

BREAKING YOUR FAST
WHEN DO YOU PLAN TO BREAK YOUR FAST?

HOW DO YOU PLAN TO BREAK YOUR FAST?

HOW DID YOU FEEL AFTER YOU BROKE YOUR FAST?

● ● ●

REFLECTION QUESTIONS

Please refer to the Questions section and select an area (or two) that resonates with you. Then choose and answer a question from the area or areas that most align with your thoughts and experiences today.

AREA OF FOCUS	MENTAL	EMOTIONAL	SPIRITUAL	PHYSICAL

QUESTION

ANSWER

Once a woman knows how to build a fasting lifestyle around her cycle, she becomes unstoppable.

"

Fasting is not
a moment of
deprivation.
It's a gift you
give yourself.

FAST TRACKING

WHAT KIND OF FAST ARE YOU DOING?

IF YOUR FAST IS LONGER THAN ONE DAY, WHAT DAY OF YOUR FAST ARE YOU ON?

(1) (2) (3) (4) (5)

KETONE LEVEL
UPON WAKING

WHAT DAY ARE YOU ON IN YOUR MENSTRUAL CYCLE?

CIRCLE THE NUMBER THAT BEST DESCRIBES HOW YOU FELT AT THE END OF TODAY'S FAST

(1) (2) (3) (4) (5)

Angry   Sad   Neutral   Happy   Overjoyed

WHAT EXERCISE/ACTIVITY HAVE YOU DONE TODAY AND HOW DID YOU FEEL WHILE DOING IT?

WHAT WENT WELL DURING YOUR FAST TODAY?

IS THERE ANYTHING YOU'D DO DIFFERENTLY?

RECORD YOUR SUGAR VALUES

UPON WAKING

MIDDAY

BEFORE BED

HOW MANY HOURS DID YOU SLEEP?

CIRCLE THE NUMBER THAT BEST DESCRIBES THE QUALITY OF YOUR SLEEP

(1) (2) (3) (4) (5)

Very Low   Low   Neutral   High   Very High

CIRCLE THE NUMBER THAT BEST DESCRIBES YOUR ENERGY LEVEL

(1) (2) (3) (4) (5)

Very Low   Low   Neutral   High   Very High

BREAKING YOUR FAST
WHEN DO YOU PLAN TO BREAK YOUR FAST?

HOW DO YOU PLAN TO BREAK YOUR FAST?

HOW DID YOU FEEL AFTER YOU BROKE YOUR FAST?

● ● ●

REFLECTION QUESTIONS

Please refer to the Questions section and select an area (or two) that resonates with you. Then choose and answer a question from the area or areas that most align with your thoughts and experiences today.

AREA OF FOCUS	MENTAL	EMOTIONAL	SPIRITUAL	PHYSICAL

QUESTION

ANSWER

FAST TRACKING

DATE ● ● ●

WHAT KIND OF FAST ARE YOU DOING?

IF YOUR FAST IS LONGER THAN ONE DAY, WHAT DAY OF YOUR FAST ARE YOU ON?

① ② ③ ④ ⑤

KETONE LEVEL
UPON WAKING

WHAT DAY ARE YOU ON IN YOUR MENSTRUAL CYCLE?

CIRCLE THE NUMBER THAT BEST DESCRIBES HOW YOU FELT AT THE END OF TODAY'S FAST

① ② ③ ④ ⑤

Angry Sad Neutral Happy Overjoyed

WHAT EXERCISE/ACTIVITY HAVE YOU DONE TODAY AND HOW DID YOU FEEL WHILE DOING IT?

WHAT WENT WELL DURING YOUR FAST TODAY?

IS THERE ANYTHING YOU'D DO DIFFERENTLY?

RECORD YOUR SUGAR VALUES

UPON WAKING

MIDDAY

BEFORE BED

HOW MANY HOURS DID YOU SLEEP?

CIRCLE THE NUMBER THAT BEST DESCRIBES THE QUALITY OF YOUR SLEEP

① ② ③ ④ ⑤

Very Low Low Neutral High Very High

CIRCLE THE NUMBER THAT BEST DESCRIBES YOUR ENERGY LEVEL

① ② ③ ④ ⑤

Very Low Low Neutral High Very High

BREAKING YOUR FAST

WHEN DO YOU PLAN TO BREAK YOUR FAST?

HOW DO YOU PLAN TO BREAK YOUR FAST?

HOW DID YOU FEEL AFTER YOU BROKE YOUR FAST?

● ● ●

REFLECTION QUESTIONS

Please refer to the Questions section and select an area (or two) that resonates with you. Then choose and answer a question from the area or areas that most align with your thoughts and experiences today.

AREA OF FOCUS	MENTAL	EMOTIONAL	SPIRITUAL	PHYSICAL

QUESTION

ANSWER

FAST TRACKING

DATE ◯ ◯ ◯

WHAT KIND OF FAST ARE YOU DOING?

IF YOUR FAST IS LONGER THAN ONE DAY, WHAT DAY OF YOUR FAST ARE YOU ON?

(1) (2) (3) (4) (5)

KETONE LEVEL
UPON WAKING

WHAT DAY ARE YOU ON IN YOUR MENSTRUAL CYCLE?

CIRCLE THE NUMBER THAT BEST DESCRIBES HOW YOU FELT AT THE END OF TODAY'S FAST

(1) (2) (3) (4) (5)

Angry   Sad   Neutral   Happy   Overjoyed

WHAT EXERCISE/ACTIVITY HAVE YOU DONE TODAY AND HOW DID YOU FEEL WHILE DOING IT?

WHAT WENT WELL DURING YOUR FAST TODAY?

IS THERE ANYTHING YOU'D DO DIFFERENTLY?

RECORD YOUR SUGAR VALUES

UPON WAKING

MIDDAY

BEFORE BED

HOW MANY HOURS DID YOU SLEEP? ◯

CIRCLE THE NUMBER THAT BEST DESCRIBES THE QUALITY OF YOUR SLEEP

(1) (2) (3) (4) (5)

Very Low   Low   Neutral   High   Very High

CIRCLE THE NUMBER THAT BEST DESCRIBES YOUR ENERGY LEVEL

(1) (2) (3) (4) (5)

Very Low   Low   Neutral   High   Very High

BREAKING YOUR FAST
WHEN DO YOU PLAN TO BREAK YOUR FAST?

HOW DO YOU PLAN TO BREAK YOUR FAST?

HOW DID YOU FEEL AFTER YOU BROKE YOUR FAST?

REFLECTION QUESTIONS

Please refer to the Questions section and select an area (or two) that resonates with you. Then choose and answer a question from the area or areas that most align with your thoughts and experiences today.

AREA OF FOCUS	MENTAL	EMOTIONAL	SPIRITUAL	PHYSICAL

QUESTION

ANSWER

FAST TRACKING

WHAT KIND OF FAST ARE YOU DOING?

IF YOUR FAST IS LONGER THAN ONE DAY, WHAT DAY OF YOUR FAST ARE YOU ON?

(1) (2) (3) (4) (5)

KETONE LEVEL
UPON WAKING

WHAT DAY ARE YOU ON IN YOUR MENSTRUAL CYCLE?

CIRCLE THE NUMBER THAT BEST DESCRIBES HOW YOU FELT AT THE END OF TODAY'S FAST

(1) (2) (3) (4) (5)

Angry   Sad   Neutral   Happy   Overjoyed

WHAT EXERCISE/ACTIVITY HAVE YOU DONE TODAY AND HOW DID YOU FEEL WHILE DOING IT?

WHAT WENT WELL DURING YOUR FAST TODAY?

IS THERE ANYTHING YOU'D DO DIFFERENTLY?

RECORD YOUR SUGAR VALUES

UPON WAKING

MIDDAY

BEFORE BED

HOW MANY HOURS DID YOU SLEEP?

CIRCLE THE NUMBER THAT BEST DESCRIBES THE QUALITY OF YOUR SLEEP

(1) (2) (3) (4) (5)

Very Low   Low   Neutral   High   Very High

CIRCLE THE NUMBER THAT BEST DESCRIBES YOUR ENERGY LEVEL

(1) (2) (3) (4) (5)

Very Low   Low   Neutral   High   Very High

BREAKING YOUR FAST
WHEN DO YOU PLAN TO BREAK YOUR FAST?

HOW DO YOU PLAN TO BREAK YOUR FAST?

HOW DID YOU FEEL AFTER YOU BROKE YOUR FAST?

● ● ●

REFLECTION QUESTIONS

Please refer to the Questions section and select an area (or two) that resonates with you. Then choose and answer a question from the area or areas that most align with your thoughts and experiences today.

AREA OF FOCUS	MENTAL	EMOTIONAL	SPIRITUAL	PHYSICAL

QUESTION

ANSWER

FAST TRACKING

DATE ◯ ◯ ◯

WHAT KIND OF FAST ARE YOU DOING?

IF YOUR FAST IS LONGER THAN ONE DAY, WHAT DAY OF YOUR FAST ARE YOU ON?

1　2　3　4　5

KETONE LEVEL
UPON WAKING

WHAT DAY ARE YOU ON IN YOUR MENSTRUAL CYCLE?

CIRCLE THE NUMBER THAT BEST DESCRIBES HOW YOU FELT AT THE END OF TODAY'S FAST

1	2	3	4	5
Angry	Sad	Neutral	Happy	Overjoyed

WHAT EXERCISE/ACTIVITY HAVE YOU DONE TODAY AND HOW DID YOU FEEL WHILE DOING IT?

WHAT WENT WELL DURING YOUR FAST TODAY?

IS THERE ANYTHING YOU'D DO DIFFERENTLY?

RECORD YOUR SUGAR VALUES

UPON WAKING

MIDDAY

BEFORE BED

HOW MANY HOURS DID YOU SLEEP? ◯

CIRCLE THE NUMBER THAT BEST DESCRIBES THE QUALITY OF YOUR SLEEP

1	2	3	4	5
Very Low	Low	Neutral	High	Very High

CIRCLE THE NUMBER THAT BEST DESCRIBES YOUR ENERGY LEVEL

1	2	3	4	5
Very Low	Low	Neutral	High	Very High

BREAKING YOUR FAST

WHEN DO YOU PLAN TO BREAK YOUR FAST?

HOW DO YOU PLAN TO BREAK YOUR FAST?

HOW DID YOU FEEL AFTER YOU BROKE YOUR FAST?

REFLECTION QUESTIONS

Please refer to the Questions section and select an area (or two) that resonates with you. Then choose and answer a question from the area or areas that most align with your thoughts and experiences today.

AREA OF FOCUS	MENTAL	EMOTIONAL	SPIRITUAL	PHYSICAL

QUESTION

ANSWER

FAST TRACKING

WHAT KIND OF FAST ARE YOU DOING?

IF YOUR FAST IS LONGER THAN ONE DAY, WHAT DAY OF YOUR FAST ARE YOU ON?

1   2   3   4   5

KETONE LEVEL
UPON WAKING

WHAT DAY ARE YOU ON IN YOUR MENSTRUAL CYCLE?

CIRCLE THE NUMBER THAT BEST DESCRIBES HOW YOU FELT AT THE END OF TODAY'S FAST

1   2   3   4   5

Angry   Sad   Neutral   Happy   Overjoyed

WHAT EXERCISE/ACTIVITY HAVE YOU DONE TODAY AND HOW DID YOU FEEL WHILE DOING IT?

WHAT WENT WELL DURING YOUR FAST TODAY?

IS THERE ANYTHING YOU'D DO DIFFERENTLY?

RECORD YOUR SUGAR VALUES

UPON WAKING

MIDDAY

BEFORE BED

HOW MANY HOURS DID YOU SLEEP?

CIRCLE THE NUMBER THAT BEST DESCRIBES THE QUALITY OF YOUR SLEEP

1   2   3   4   5

Very Low   Low   Neutral   High   Very High

CIRCLE THE NUMBER THAT BEST DESCRIBES YOUR ENERGY LEVEL

1   2   3   4   5

Very Low   Low   Neutral   High   Very High

BREAKING YOUR FAST

WHEN DO YOU PLAN TO BREAK YOUR FAST?

HOW DO YOU PLAN TO BREAK YOUR FAST?

HOW DID YOU FEEL AFTER YOU BROKE YOUR FAST?

REFLECTION QUESTIONS

Please refer to the Questions section and select an area (or two) that resonates with you. Then choose and answer a question from the area or areas that most align with your thoughts and experiences today.

AREA OF FOCUS	MENTAL	EMOTIONAL	SPIRITUAL	PHYSICAL

QUESTION

ANSWER

> Fasting allows your body and brain to recover from the stressors of the modern world.

66

The results you've
been searching for
through dieting can
now be achieved
through fasting.

FAST TRACKING

WHAT KIND OF FAST ARE YOU DOING?

IF YOUR FAST IS LONGER THAN ONE DAY, WHAT DAY OF YOUR FAST ARE YOU ON?

1   2   3   4   5

KETONE LEVEL
UPON WAKING

WHAT DAY ARE YOU ON IN YOUR MENSTRUAL CYCLE?

CIRCLE THE NUMBER THAT BEST DESCRIBES HOW YOU FELT AT THE END OF TODAY'S FAST

1   2   3   4   5
Angry   Sad   Neutral   Happy   Overjoyed

WHAT EXERCISE/ACTIVITY HAVE YOU DONE TODAY AND HOW DID YOU FEEL WHILE DOING IT?

WHAT WENT WELL DURING YOUR FAST TODAY?

IS THERE ANYTHING YOU'D DO DIFFERENTLY?

RECORD YOUR SUGAR VALUES

UPON WAKING

MIDDAY

BEFORE BED

HOW MANY HOURS DID YOU SLEEP?

CIRCLE THE NUMBER THAT BEST DESCRIBES THE QUALITY OF YOUR SLEEP

1   2   3   4   5
Very Low   Low   Neutral   High   Very High

CIRCLE THE NUMBER THAT BEST DESCRIBES YOUR ENERGY LEVEL

1   2   3   4   5
Very Low   Low   Neutral   High   Very High

BREAKING YOUR FAST
WHEN DO YOU PLAN TO BREAK YOUR FAST?

HOW DO YOU PLAN TO BREAK YOUR FAST?

HOW DID YOU FEEL AFTER YOU BROKE YOUR FAST?

● ● ●

REFLECTION QUESTIONS

Please refer to the Questions section and select an area (or two) that resonates with you. Then choose and answer a question from the area or areas that most align with your thoughts and experiences today.

AREA OF FOCUS	MENTAL	EMOTIONAL	SPIRITUAL	PHYSICAL

QUESTION

ANSWER

FAST TRACKING

WHAT KIND OF FAST ARE YOU DOING?

IF YOUR FAST IS LONGER THAN ONE DAY, WHAT DAY OF YOUR FAST ARE YOU ON?

1   2   3   4   5

KETONE LEVEL
UPON WAKING

WHAT DAY ARE YOU ON IN YOUR MENSTRUAL CYCLE?

CIRCLE THE NUMBER THAT BEST DESCRIBES HOW YOU FELT AT THE END OF TODAY'S FAST

1	2	3	4	5
Angry	Sad	Neutral	Happy	Overjoyed

WHAT EXERCISE/ACTIVITY HAVE YOU DONE TODAY AND HOW DID YOU FEEL WHILE DOING IT?

WHAT WENT WELL DURING YOUR FAST TODAY?

IS THERE ANYTHING YOU'D DO DIFFERENTLY?

RECORD YOUR SUGAR VALUES

UPON WAKING

MIDDAY

BEFORE BED

HOW MANY HOURS DID YOU SLEEP?

CIRCLE THE NUMBER THAT BEST DESCRIBES THE QUALITY OF YOUR SLEEP

1	2	3	4	5
Very Low	Low	Neutral	High	Very High

CIRCLE THE NUMBER THAT BEST DESCRIBES YOUR ENERGY LEVEL

1	2	3	4	5
Very Low	Low	Neutral	High	Very High

BREAKING YOUR FAST

WHEN DO YOU PLAN TO BREAK YOUR FAST?

HOW DO YOU PLAN TO BREAK YOUR FAST?

HOW DID YOU FEEL AFTER YOU BROKE YOUR FAST?

REFLECTION QUESTIONS

Please refer to the Questions section and select an area (or two) that resonates with you. Then choose and answer a question from the area or areas that most align with your thoughts and experiences today.

AREA OF FOCUS	MENTAL	EMOTIONAL	SPIRITUAL	PHYSICAL

QUESTION

ANSWER

● ● ●

FAST TRACKING

WHAT KIND OF FAST ARE YOU DOING?

IF YOUR FAST IS LONGER THAN ONE DAY, WHAT DAY OF YOUR FAST ARE YOU ON?

1   2   3   4   5

KETONE LEVEL
UPON WAKING

WHAT DAY ARE YOU ON IN YOUR MENSTRUAL CYCLE?

CIRCLE THE NUMBER THAT BEST DESCRIBES HOW YOU FELT AT THE END OF TODAY'S FAST

1	2	3	4	5
Angry	Sad	Neutral	Happy	Overjoyed

WHAT EXERCISE/ACTIVITY HAVE YOU DONE TODAY AND HOW DID YOU FEEL WHILE DOING IT?

WHAT WENT WELL DURING YOUR FAST TODAY?

IS THERE ANYTHING YOU'D DO DIFFERENTLY?

RECORD YOUR SUGAR VALUES

UPON WAKING

MIDDAY

BEFORE BED

HOW MANY HOURS DID YOU SLEEP?

CIRCLE THE NUMBER THAT BEST DESCRIBES THE QUALITY OF YOUR SLEEP

1	2	3	4	5
Very Low	Low	Neutral	High	Very High

CIRCLE THE NUMBER THAT BEST DESCRIBES YOUR ENERGY LEVEL

1	2	3	4	5
Very Low	Low	Neutral	High	Very High

BREAKING YOUR FAST
WHEN DO YOU PLAN TO BREAK YOUR FAST?

HOW DO YOU PLAN TO BREAK YOUR FAST?

HOW DID YOU FEEL AFTER YOU BROKE YOUR FAST?

● ● ●

REFLECTION QUESTIONS

Please refer to the Questions section and select an area (or two) that resonates with you. Then choose and answer a question from the area or areas that most align with your thoughts and experiences today.

AREA OF FOCUS	MENTAL	EMOTIONAL	SPIRITUAL	PHYSICAL

QUESTION

ANSWER

FAST TRACKING

WHAT KIND OF FAST ARE YOU DOING?

IF YOUR FAST IS LONGER THAN ONE DAY, WHAT DAY OF YOUR FAST ARE YOU ON?

1   2   3   4   5

KETONE LEVEL
UPON WAKING

WHAT DAY ARE YOU ON IN YOUR MENSTRUAL CYCLE?

CIRCLE THE NUMBER THAT BEST DESCRIBES HOW YOU FELT AT THE END OF TODAY'S FAST

1   2   3   4   5

Angry   Sad   Neutral   Happy   Overjoyed

WHAT EXERCISE/ACTIVITY HAVE YOU DONE TODAY AND HOW DID YOU FEEL WHILE DOING IT?

WHAT WENT WELL DURING YOUR FAST TODAY?

IS THERE ANYTHING YOU'D DO DIFFERENTLY?

RECORD YOUR SUGAR VALUES
UPON WAKING

MIDDAY

BEFORE BED

HOW MANY HOURS DID YOU SLEEP?

CIRCLE THE NUMBER THAT BEST DESCRIBES THE QUALITY OF YOUR SLEEP

1   2   3   4   5

Very Low   Low   Neutral   High   Very High

CIRCLE THE NUMBER THAT BEST DESCRIBES YOUR ENERGY LEVEL

1   2   3   4   5

Very Low   Low   Neutral   High   Very High

BREAKING YOUR FAST
WHEN DO YOU PLAN TO BREAK YOUR FAST?

HOW DO YOU PLAN TO BREAK YOUR FAST?

HOW DID YOU FEEL AFTER YOU BROKE YOUR FAST?

REFLECTION QUESTIONS

Please refer to the Questions section and select an area (or two) that resonates with you. Then choose and answer a question from the area or areas that most align with your thoughts and experiences today.

AREA OF FOCUS	MENTAL	EMOTIONAL	SPIRITUAL	PHYSICAL

QUESTION

ANSWER

FAST TRACKING

WHAT KIND OF FAST ARE YOU DOING?

IF YOUR FAST IS LONGER THAN ONE DAY, WHAT DAY OF YOUR FAST ARE YOU ON?

1   2   3   4   5

KETONE LEVEL
UPON WAKING

WHAT DAY ARE YOU ON IN YOUR MENSTRUAL CYCLE?

CIRCLE THE NUMBER THAT BEST DESCRIBES HOW YOU FELT AT THE END OF TODAY'S FAST

1   2   3   4   5

Angry   Sad   Neutral   Happy   Overjoyed

WHAT EXERCISE/ACTIVITY HAVE YOU DONE TODAY AND HOW DID YOU FEEL WHILE DOING IT?

WHAT WENT WELL DURING YOUR FAST TODAY?

IS THERE ANYTHING YOU'D DO DIFFERENTLY?

RECORD YOUR SUGAR VALUES

UPON WAKING

MIDDAY

BEFORE BED

HOW MANY HOURS DID YOU SLEEP?

CIRCLE THE NUMBER THAT BEST DESCRIBES THE QUALITY OF YOUR SLEEP

1   2   3   4   5

Very Low   Low   Neutral   High   Very High

CIRCLE THE NUMBER THAT BEST DESCRIBES YOUR ENERGY LEVEL

1   2   3   4   5

Very Low   Low   Neutral   High   Very High

BREAKING YOUR FAST
WHEN DO YOU PLAN TO BREAK YOUR FAST?

HOW DO YOU PLAN TO BREAK YOUR FAST?

HOW DID YOU FEEL AFTER YOU BROKE YOUR FAST?

REFLECTION QUESTIONS

Please refer to the Questions section and select an area (or two) that resonates with you. Then choose and answer a question from the area or areas that most align with your thoughts and experiences today.

AREA OF FOCUS	MENTAL	EMOTIONAL	SPIRITUAL	PHYSICAL

QUESTION

ANSWER

FAST TRACKING

WHAT KIND OF FAST ARE YOU DOING?

IF YOUR FAST IS LONGER THAN ONE DAY, WHAT DAY OF YOUR FAST ARE YOU ON?

1   2   3   4   5

KETONE LEVEL
UPON WAKING

WHAT DAY ARE YOU ON IN YOUR MENSTRUAL CYCLE?

CIRCLE THE NUMBER THAT BEST DESCRIBES HOW YOU FELT AT THE END OF TODAY'S FAST

1   2   3   4   5
Angry   Sad   Neutral   Happy   Overjoyed

WHAT EXERCISE/ACTIVITY HAVE YOU DONE TODAY AND HOW DID YOU FEEL WHILE DOING IT?

WHAT WENT WELL DURING YOUR FAST TODAY?

IS THERE ANYTHING YOU'D DO DIFFERENTLY?

RECORD YOUR SUGAR VALUES

UPON WAKING

MIDDAY

BEFORE BED

HOW MANY HOURS DID YOU SLEEP? ◯

CIRCLE THE NUMBER THAT BEST DESCRIBES THE QUALITY OF YOUR SLEEP

1   2   3   4   5
Very Low   Low   Neutral   High   Very High

CIRCLE THE NUMBER THAT BEST DESCRIBES YOUR ENERGY LEVEL

1   2   3   4   5
Very Low   Low   Neutral   High   Very High

BREAKING YOUR FAST
WHEN DO YOU PLAN TO BREAK YOUR FAST?

HOW DO YOU PLAN TO BREAK YOUR FAST?

HOW DID YOU FEEL AFTER YOU BROKE YOUR FAST?

• • •

REFLECTION QUESTIONS

Please refer to the Questions section and select an area (or two) that resonates with you. Then choose and answer a question from the area or areas that most align with your thoughts and experiences today.

AREA OF FOCUS	MENTAL	EMOTIONAL	SPIRITUAL	PHYSICAL

QUESTION

ANSWER

" You are the
miracle, not
the diet.

"

You are powerful
beyond your wildest
imagination. Starting
now, you can step
into a new possibility.

FAST TRACKING

WHAT KIND OF FAST ARE YOU DOING?

IF YOUR FAST IS LONGER THAN ONE DAY, WHAT DAY OF YOUR FAST ARE YOU ON?

(1) (2) (3) (4) (5)

KETONE LEVEL
UPON WAKING

WHAT DAY ARE YOU ON IN YOUR MENSTRUAL CYCLE?

CIRCLE THE NUMBER THAT BEST DESCRIBES HOW YOU FELT AT THE END OF TODAY'S FAST

(1) (2) (3) (4) (5)

Angry   Sad   Neutral   Happy   Overjoyed

WHAT EXERCISE/ACTIVITY HAVE YOU DONE TODAY AND HOW DID YOU FEEL WHILE DOING IT?

WHAT WENT WELL DURING YOUR FAST TODAY?

IS THERE ANYTHING YOU'D DO DIFFERENTLY?

RECORD YOUR SUGAR VALUES

UPON WAKING

MIDDAY

BEFORE BED

HOW MANY HOURS DID YOU SLEEP?

CIRCLE THE NUMBER THAT BEST DESCRIBES THE QUALITY OF YOUR SLEEP

(1) (2) (3) (4) (5)

Very Low   Low   Neutral   High   Very High

CIRCLE THE NUMBER THAT BEST DESCRIBES YOUR ENERGY LEVEL

(1) (2) (3) (4) (5)

Very Low   Low   Neutral   High   Very High

BREAKING YOUR FAST
WHEN DO YOU PLAN TO BREAK YOUR FAST?

HOW DO YOU PLAN TO BREAK YOUR FAST?

HOW DID YOU FEEL AFTER YOU BROKE YOUR FAST?

REFLECTION QUESTIONS

Please refer to the Questions section and select an area (or two) that resonates with you. Then choose and answer a question from the area or areas that most align with your thoughts and experiences today.

AREA OF FOCUS	MENTAL	EMOTIONAL	SPIRITUAL	PHYSICAL

QUESTION

ANSWER

FAST TRACKING

WHAT KIND OF FAST ARE YOU DOING?

IF YOUR FAST IS LONGER THAN ONE DAY, WHAT DAY OF YOUR FAST ARE YOU ON?

(1) (2) (3) (4) (5)

KETONE LEVEL
UPON WAKING

WHAT DAY ARE YOU ON IN YOUR MENSTRUAL CYCLE?

CIRCLE THE NUMBER THAT BEST DESCRIBES HOW YOU FELT AT THE END OF TODAY'S FAST

(1) (2) (3) (4) (5)
Angry Sad Neutral Happy Overjoyed

WHAT EXERCISE/ACTIVITY HAVE YOU DONE TODAY AND HOW DID YOU FEEL WHILE DOING IT?

WHAT WENT WELL DURING YOUR FAST TODAY?

IS THERE ANYTHING YOU'D DO DIFFERENTLY?

RECORD YOUR SUGAR VALUES

UPON WAKING

MIDDAY

BEFORE BED

HOW MANY HOURS DID YOU SLEEP? ◯

CIRCLE THE NUMBER THAT BEST DESCRIBES THE QUALITY OF YOUR SLEEP

(1) (2) (3) (4) (5)
Very Low Low Neutral High Very High

CIRCLE THE NUMBER THAT BEST DESCRIBES YOUR ENERGY LEVEL

(1) (2) (3) (4) (5)
Very Low Low Neutral High Very High

BREAKING YOUR FAST
WHEN DO YOU PLAN TO BREAK YOUR FAST?

HOW DO YOU PLAN TO BREAK YOUR FAST?

HOW DID YOU FEEL AFTER YOU BROKE YOUR FAST?

REFLECTION QUESTIONS

Please refer to the Questions section and select an area (or two) that resonates with you. Then choose and answer a question from the area or areas that most align with your thoughts and experiences today.

AREA OF FOCUS	MENTAL	EMOTIONAL	SPIRITUAL	PHYSICAL

QUESTION

ANSWER

FAST TRACKING

DATE ◯ ◯ ◯

WHAT KIND OF FAST ARE YOU DOING?

IF YOUR FAST IS LONGER THAN ONE DAY, WHAT DAY OF YOUR FAST ARE YOU ON?

(1) (2) (3) (4) (5)

KETONE LEVEL
UPON WAKING

WHAT DAY ARE YOU ON IN YOUR MENSTRUAL CYCLE?

CIRCLE THE NUMBER THAT BEST DESCRIBES HOW YOU FELT AT THE END OF TODAY'S FAST

(1) (2) (3) (4) (5)

Angry   Sad   Neutral   Happy   Overjoyed

WHAT EXERCISE/ACTIVITY HAVE YOU DONE TODAY AND HOW DID YOU FEEL WHILE DOING IT?

WHAT WENT WELL DURING YOUR FAST TODAY?

IS THERE ANYTHING YOU'D DO DIFFERENTLY?

RECORD YOUR SUGAR VALUES

UPON WAKING

MIDDAY

BEFORE BED

HOW MANY HOURS DID YOU SLEEP? ◯

CIRCLE THE NUMBER THAT BEST DESCRIBES THE QUALITY OF YOUR SLEEP

(1) (2) (3) (4) (5)

Very Low   Low   Neutral   High   Very High

CIRCLE THE NUMBER THAT BEST DESCRIBES YOUR ENERGY LEVEL

(1) (2) (3) (4) (5)

Very Low   Low   Neutral   High   Very High

BREAKING YOUR FAST
WHEN DO YOU PLAN TO BREAK YOUR FAST?

HOW DO YOU PLAN TO BREAK YOUR FAST?

HOW DID YOU FEEL AFTER YOU BROKE YOUR FAST?

● ● ●

REFLECTION QUESTIONS

Please refer to the Questions section and select an area (or two) that resonates with you. Then choose and answer a question from the area or areas that most align with your thoughts and experiences today.

AREA OF FOCUS	MENTAL	EMOTIONAL	SPIRITUAL	PHYSICAL

QUESTION

ANSWER

FAST TRACKING

WHAT KIND OF FAST ARE YOU DOING?

IF YOUR FAST IS LONGER THAN ONE DAY, WHAT DAY OF YOUR FAST ARE YOU ON?

1   2   3   4   5

RECORD YOUR SUGAR VALUES

UPON WAKING

MIDDAY

BEFORE BED

KETONE LEVEL
UPON WAKING

WHAT DAY ARE YOU ON IN YOUR MENSTRUAL CYCLE?

HOW MANY HOURS DID YOU SLEEP? ◯

CIRCLE THE NUMBER THAT BEST DESCRIBES THE QUALITY OF YOUR SLEEP

1   2   3   4   5
Very Low   Low   Neutral   High   Very High

CIRCLE THE NUMBER THAT BEST DESCRIBES HOW YOU FELT AT THE END OF TODAY'S FAST

1   2   3   4   5
Angry   Sad   Neutral   Happy   Overjoyed

CIRCLE THE NUMBER THAT BEST DESCRIBES YOUR ENERGY LEVEL

1   2   3   4   5
Very Low   Low   Neutral   High   Very High

WHAT EXERCISE/ACTIVITY HAVE YOU DONE TODAY AND HOW DID YOU FEEL WHILE DOING IT?

WHAT WENT WELL DURING YOUR FAST TODAY?

IS THERE ANYTHING YOU'D DO DIFFERENTLY?

BREAKING YOUR FAST
WHEN DO YOU PLAN TO BREAK YOUR FAST?

HOW DO YOU PLAN TO BREAK YOUR FAST?

HOW DID YOU FEEL AFTER YOU BROKE YOUR FAST?

REFLECTION QUESTIONS

Please refer to the Questions section and select an area (or two) that resonates with you. Then choose and answer a question from the area or areas that most align with your thoughts and experiences today.

AREA OF FOCUS	MENTAL	EMOTIONAL	SPIRITUAL	PHYSICAL

QUESTION

ANSWER

FAST TRACKING

WHAT KIND OF FAST ARE YOU DOING?

IF YOUR FAST IS LONGER THAN ONE DAY, WHAT DAY OF YOUR FAST ARE YOU ON?

(1) (2) (3) (4) (5)

KETONE LEVEL
UPON WAKING

WHAT DAY ARE YOU ON IN YOUR MENSTRUAL CYCLE?

CIRCLE THE NUMBER THAT BEST DESCRIBES HOW YOU FELT AT THE END OF TODAY'S FAST

(1) (2) (3) (4) (5)

Angry   Sad   Neutral   Happy   Overjoyed

WHAT EXERCISE/ACTIVITY HAVE YOU DONE TODAY AND HOW DID YOU FEEL WHILE DOING IT?

WHAT WENT WELL DURING YOUR FAST TODAY?

IS THERE ANYTHING YOU'D DO DIFFERENTLY?

RECORD YOUR SUGAR VALUES

UPON WAKING

MIDDAY

BEFORE BED

HOW MANY HOURS DID YOU SLEEP? ◯

CIRCLE THE NUMBER THAT BEST DESCRIBES THE QUALITY OF YOUR SLEEP

(1) (2) (3) (4) (5)

Very Low   Low   Neutral   High   Very High

CIRCLE THE NUMBER THAT BEST DESCRIBES YOUR ENERGY LEVEL

(1) (2) (3) (4) (5)

Very Low   Low   Neutral   High   Very High

BREAKING YOUR FAST
WHEN DO YOU PLAN TO BREAK YOUR FAST?

HOW DO YOU PLAN TO BREAK YOUR FAST?

HOW DID YOU FEEL AFTER YOU BROKE YOUR FAST?

REFLECTION QUESTIONS

Please refer to the Questions section and select an area (or two) that resonates with you. Then choose and answer a question from the area or areas that most align with your thoughts and experiences today.

AREA OF FOCUS	MENTAL	EMOTIONAL	SPIRITUAL	PHYSICAL

QUESTION

ANSWER

FAST TRACKING

WHAT KIND OF FAST ARE YOU DOING?

IF YOUR FAST IS LONGER THAN ONE DAY, WHAT DAY OF YOUR FAST ARE YOU ON?

(1) (2) (3) (4) (5)

KETONE LEVEL
UPON WAKING

WHAT DAY ARE YOU ON IN YOUR MENSTRUAL CYCLE?

CIRCLE THE NUMBER THAT BEST DESCRIBES HOW YOU FELT AT THE END OF TODAY'S FAST

(1)	(2)	(3)	(4)	(5)
Angry	Sad	Neutral	Happy	Overjoyed

WHAT EXERCISE/ACTIVITY HAVE YOU DONE TODAY AND HOW DID YOU FEEL WHILE DOING IT?

WHAT WENT WELL DURING YOUR FAST TODAY?

IS THERE ANYTHING YOU'D DO DIFFERENTLY?

RECORD YOUR SUGAR VALUES

UPON WAKING

MIDDAY

BEFORE BED

HOW MANY HOURS DID YOU SLEEP? ◯

CIRCLE THE NUMBER THAT BEST DESCRIBES THE QUALITY OF YOUR SLEEP

(1)	(2)	(3)	(4)	(5)
Very Low	Low	Neutral	High	Very High

CIRCLE THE NUMBER THAT BEST DESCRIBES YOUR ENERGY LEVEL

(1)	(2)	(3)	(4)	(5)
Very Low	Low	Neutral	High	Very High

BREAKING YOUR FAST

WHEN DO YOU PLAN TO BREAK YOUR FAST?

HOW DO YOU PLAN TO BREAK YOUR FAST?

HOW DID YOU FEEL AFTER YOU BROKE YOUR FAST?

REFLECTION QUESTIONS

Please refer to the Questions section and select an area (or two) that resonates with you. Then choose and answer a question from the area or areas that most align with your thoughts and experiences today.

AREA OF FOCUS	MENTAL	EMOTIONAL	SPIRITUAL	PHYSICAL

QUESTION

ANSWER

One of the amazing
things about
your body is that
it is constantly
regenerating itself.

66 ——

The number one
goal for your
health should be
loving the body
you are living in.

FAST TRACKING

WHAT KIND OF FAST ARE YOU DOING?

IF YOUR FAST IS LONGER THAN ONE DAY, WHAT DAY OF YOUR FAST ARE YOU ON?

1   2   3   4   5

KETONE LEVEL
UPON WAKING

WHAT DAY ARE YOU ON IN YOUR MENSTRUAL CYCLE?

CIRCLE THE NUMBER THAT BEST DESCRIBES HOW YOU FELT AT THE END OF TODAY'S FAST

1   2   3   4   5

Angry   Sad   Neutral   Happy   Overjoyed

WHAT EXERCISE/ACTIVITY HAVE YOU DONE TODAY AND HOW DID YOU FEEL WHILE DOING IT?

WHAT WENT WELL DURING YOUR FAST TODAY?

IS THERE ANYTHING YOU'D DO DIFFERENTLY?

RECORD YOUR SUGAR VALUES

UPON WAKING

MIDDAY

BEFORE BED

HOW MANY HOURS DID YOU SLEEP?

CIRCLE THE NUMBER THAT BEST DESCRIBES THE QUALITY OF YOUR SLEEP

1   2   3   4   5

Very Low   Low   Neutral   High   Very High

CIRCLE THE NUMBER THAT BEST DESCRIBES YOUR ENERGY LEVEL

1   2   3   4   5

Very Low   Low   Neutral   High   Very High

BREAKING YOUR FAST
WHEN DO YOU PLAN TO BREAK YOUR FAST?

HOW DO YOU PLAN TO BREAK YOUR FAST?

HOW DID YOU FEEL AFTER YOU BROKE YOUR FAST?

REFLECTION QUESTIONS

Please refer to the Questions section and select an area (or two) that resonates with you. Then choose and answer a question from the area or areas that most align with your thoughts and experiences today.

| AREA OF FOCUS | MENTAL | EMOTIONAL | SPIRITUAL | PHYSICAL |

QUESTION

ANSWER

FAST TRACKING

WHAT KIND OF FAST ARE YOU DOING?

IF YOUR FAST IS LONGER THAN ONE DAY, WHAT DAY OF YOUR FAST ARE YOU ON?

1 2 3 4 5

KETONE LEVEL
UPON WAKING

WHAT DAY ARE YOU ON IN YOUR MENSTRUAL CYCLE?

CIRCLE THE NUMBER THAT BEST DESCRIBES HOW YOU FELT AT THE END OF TODAY'S FAST

1 2 3 4 5

Angry Sad Neutral Happy Overjoyed

WHAT EXERCISE/ACTIVITY HAVE YOU DONE TODAY AND HOW DID YOU FEEL WHILE DOING IT?

WHAT WENT WELL DURING YOUR FAST TODAY?

IS THERE ANYTHING YOU'D DO DIFFERENTLY?

RECORD YOUR SUGAR VALUES

UPON WAKING

MIDDAY

BEFORE BED

HOW MANY HOURS DID YOU SLEEP?

CIRCLE THE NUMBER THAT BEST DESCRIBES THE QUALITY OF YOUR SLEEP

1 2 3 4 5

Very Low Low Neutral High Very High

CIRCLE THE NUMBER THAT BEST DESCRIBES YOUR ENERGY LEVEL

1 2 3 4 5

Very Low Low Neutral High Very High

BREAKING YOUR FAST

WHEN DO YOU PLAN TO BREAK YOUR FAST?

HOW DO YOU PLAN TO BREAK YOUR FAST?

HOW DID YOU FEEL AFTER YOU BROKE YOUR FAST?

REFLECTION QUESTIONS

Please refer to the Questions section and select an area (or two) that resonates with you. Then choose and answer a question from the area or areas that most align with your thoughts and experiences today.

AREA OF FOCUS	MENTAL	EMOTIONAL	SPIRITUAL	PHYSICAL

QUESTION

ANSWER

FAST TRACKING

WHAT KIND OF FAST ARE YOU DOING?

IF YOUR FAST IS LONGER THAN ONE DAY, WHAT DAY OF YOUR FAST ARE YOU ON?

1   2   3   4   5

KETONE LEVEL
UPON WAKING

WHAT DAY ARE YOU ON IN YOUR MENSTRUAL CYCLE?

CIRCLE THE NUMBER THAT BEST DESCRIBES HOW YOU FELT AT THE END OF TODAY'S FAST

1   2   3   4   5

Angry   Sad   Neutral   Happy   Overjoyed

WHAT EXERCISE/ACTIVITY HAVE YOU DONE TODAY AND HOW DID YOU FEEL WHILE DOING IT?

WHAT WENT WELL DURING YOUR FAST TODAY?

IS THERE ANYTHING YOU'D DO DIFFERENTLY?

RECORD YOUR SUGAR VALUES

UPON WAKING

MIDDAY

BEFORE BED

HOW MANY HOURS DID YOU SLEEP?

CIRCLE THE NUMBER THAT BEST DESCRIBES THE QUALITY OF YOUR SLEEP

1   2   3   4   5

Very Low   Low   Neutral   High   Very High

CIRCLE THE NUMBER THAT BEST DESCRIBES YOUR ENERGY LEVEL

1   2   3   4   5

Very Low   Low   Neutral   High   Very High

BREAKING YOUR FAST

WHEN DO YOU PLAN TO BREAK YOUR FAST?

HOW DO YOU PLAN TO BREAK YOUR FAST?

HOW DID YOU FEEL AFTER YOU BROKE YOUR FAST?

● ● ●

REFLECTION QUESTIONS

Please refer to the Questions section and select an area (or two) that resonates with you. Then choose and answer a question from the area or areas that most align with your thoughts and experiences today.

AREA OF FOCUS	MENTAL	EMOTIONAL	SPIRITUAL	PHYSICAL

QUESTION

ANSWER

FAST TRACKING

WHAT KIND OF FAST ARE YOU DOING?

IF YOUR FAST IS LONGER THAN ONE DAY, WHAT DAY OF YOUR FAST ARE YOU ON?

1   2   3   4   5

KETONE LEVEL
UPON WAKING

WHAT DAY ARE YOU ON IN YOUR MENSTRUAL CYCLE?

CIRCLE THE NUMBER THAT BEST DESCRIBES HOW YOU FELT AT THE END OF TODAY'S FAST

1   2   3   4   5

Angry   Sad   Neutral   Happy   Overjoyed

WHAT EXERCISE/ACTIVITY HAVE YOU DONE TODAY AND HOW DID YOU FEEL WHILE DOING IT?

WHAT WENT WELL DURING YOUR FAST TODAY?

IS THERE ANYTHING YOU'D DO DIFFERENTLY?

RECORD YOUR SUGAR VALUES

UPON WAKING

MIDDAY

BEFORE BED

HOW MANY HOURS DID YOU SLEEP?

CIRCLE THE NUMBER THAT BEST DESCRIBES THE QUALITY OF YOUR SLEEP

1   2   3   4   5

Very Low   Low   Neutral   High   Very High

CIRCLE THE NUMBER THAT BEST DESCRIBES YOUR ENERGY LEVEL

1   2   3   4   5

Very Low   Low   Neutral   High   Very High

BREAKING YOUR FAST
WHEN DO YOU PLAN TO BREAK YOUR FAST?

HOW DO YOU PLAN TO BREAK YOUR FAST?

HOW DID YOU FEEL AFTER YOU BROKE YOUR FAST?

REFLECTION QUESTIONS

Please refer to the Questions section and select an area (or two) that resonates with you. Then choose and answer a question from the area or areas that most align with your thoughts and experiences today.

AREA OF FOCUS	MENTAL	EMOTIONAL	SPIRITUAL	PHYSICAL

QUESTION

ANSWER

FAST TRACKING

WHAT KIND OF FAST ARE YOU DOING?

IF YOUR FAST IS LONGER THAN ONE DAY, WHAT DAY OF YOUR FAST ARE YOU ON?

1   2   3   4   5

KETONE LEVEL
UPON WAKING

WHAT DAY ARE YOU ON IN YOUR MENSTRUAL CYCLE?

CIRCLE THE NUMBER THAT BEST DESCRIBES HOW YOU FELT AT THE END OF TODAY'S FAST

1   2   3   4   5

Angry   Sad   Neutral   Happy   Overjoyed

WHAT EXERCISE/ACTIVITY HAVE YOU DONE TODAY AND HOW DID YOU FEEL WHILE DOING IT?

WHAT WENT WELL DURING YOUR FAST TODAY?

IS THERE ANYTHING YOU'D DO DIFFERENTLY?

RECORD YOUR SUGAR VALUES

UPON WAKING

MIDDAY

BEFORE BED

HOW MANY HOURS DID YOU SLEEP?

CIRCLE THE NUMBER THAT BEST DESCRIBES THE QUALITY OF YOUR SLEEP

1   2   3   4   5

Very Low   Low   Neutral   High   Very High

CIRCLE THE NUMBER THAT BEST DESCRIBES YOUR ENERGY LEVEL

1   2   3   4   5

Very Low   Low   Neutral   High   Very High

BREAKING YOUR FAST

WHEN DO YOU PLAN TO BREAK YOUR FAST?

HOW DO YOU PLAN TO BREAK YOUR FAST?

HOW DID YOU FEEL AFTER YOU BROKE YOUR FAST?

● ● ●

REFLECTION QUESTIONS

Please refer to the Questions section and select an area (or two) that resonates with you. Then choose and answer a question from the area or areas that most align with your thoughts and experiences today.

AREA OF FOCUS	MENTAL	EMOTIONAL	SPIRITUAL	PHYSICAL

QUESTION

ANSWER

FAST TRACKING

WHAT KIND OF FAST ARE YOU DOING?

IF YOUR FAST IS LONGER THAN ONE DAY, WHAT DAY OF YOUR FAST ARE YOU ON?

1   2   3   4   5

KETONE LEVEL
UPON WAKING

WHAT DAY ARE YOU ON IN YOUR MENSTRUAL CYCLE?

CIRCLE THE NUMBER THAT BEST DESCRIBES HOW YOU FELT AT THE END OF TODAY'S FAST

1	2	3	4	5
Angry	Sad	Neutral	Happy	Overjoyed

WHAT EXERCISE/ACTIVITY HAVE YOU DONE TODAY AND HOW DID YOU FEEL WHILE DOING IT?

WHAT WENT WELL DURING YOUR FAST TODAY?

IS THERE ANYTHING YOU'D DO DIFFERENTLY?

RECORD YOUR SUGAR VALUES

UPON WAKING

MIDDAY

BEFORE BED

HOW MANY HOURS DID YOU SLEEP?

CIRCLE THE NUMBER THAT BEST DESCRIBES THE QUALITY OF YOUR SLEEP

1	2	3	4	5
Very Low	Low	Neutral	High	Very High

CIRCLE THE NUMBER THAT BEST DESCRIBES YOUR ENERGY LEVEL

1	2	3	4	5
Very Low	Low	Neutral	High	Very High

BREAKING YOUR FAST

WHEN DO YOU PLAN TO BREAK YOUR FAST?

HOW DO YOU PLAN TO BREAK YOUR FAST?

HOW DID YOU FEEL AFTER YOU BROKE YOUR FAST?

REFLECTION QUESTIONS

Please refer to the Questions section and select an area (or two) that resonates with you. Then choose and answer a question from the area or areas that most align with your thoughts and experiences today.

AREA OF FOCUS	MENTAL	EMOTIONAL	SPIRITUAL	PHYSICAL

QUESTION

ANSWER

> **If you don't make time for your WELLNESS, you will be forced to take time for your ILLNESS.**

66

Fasting is a
healing state that
your body wants
to thrive in.

FAST TRACKING

DATE ◯ ◯ ◯

WHAT KIND OF FAST ARE YOU DOING?

IF YOUR FAST IS LONGER THAN ONE DAY, WHAT DAY OF YOUR FAST ARE YOU ON?

1   2   3   4   5

KETONE LEVEL
UPON WAKING

WHAT DAY ARE YOU ON IN YOUR MENSTRUAL CYCLE?

CIRCLE THE NUMBER THAT BEST DESCRIBES HOW YOU FELT AT THE END OF TODAY'S FAST

1	2	3	4	5
Angry	Sad	Neutral	Happy	Overjoyed

WHAT EXERCISE/ACTIVITY HAVE YOU DONE TODAY AND HOW DID YOU FEEL WHILE DOING IT?

WHAT WENT WELL DURING YOUR FAST TODAY?

IS THERE ANYTHING YOU'D DO DIFFERENTLY?

RECORD YOUR SUGAR VALUES

UPON WAKING

MIDDAY

BEFORE BED

HOW MANY HOURS DID YOU SLEEP?

CIRCLE THE NUMBER THAT BEST DESCRIBES THE QUALITY OF YOUR SLEEP

1	2	3	4	5
Very Low	Low	Neutral	High	Very High

CIRCLE THE NUMBER THAT BEST DESCRIBES YOUR ENERGY LEVEL

1	2	3	4	5
Very Low	Low	Neutral	High	Very High

BREAKING YOUR FAST

WHEN DO YOU PLAN TO BREAK YOUR FAST?

HOW DO YOU PLAN TO BREAK YOUR FAST?

HOW DID YOU FEEL AFTER YOU BROKE YOUR FAST?

• • •

REFLECTION QUESTIONS

Please refer to the Questions section and select an area (or two) that resonates with you. Then choose and answer a question from the area or areas that most align with your thoughts and experiences today.

| AREA OF FOCUS | MENTAL | EMOTIONAL | SPIRITUAL | PHYSICAL |

QUESTION

ANSWER

FAST TRACKING

DATE ◯ ◯ ◯

WHAT KIND OF FAST ARE YOU DOING?

IF YOUR FAST IS LONGER THAN ONE DAY, WHAT DAY OF YOUR FAST ARE YOU ON?

1   2   3   4   5

KETONE LEVEL
UPON WAKING

WHAT DAY ARE YOU ON IN YOUR MENSTRUAL CYCLE?

CIRCLE THE NUMBER THAT BEST DESCRIBES HOW YOU FELT AT THE END OF TODAY'S FAST

1   2   3   4   5

Angry   Sad   Neutral   Happy   Overjoyed

WHAT EXERCISE/ACTIVITY HAVE YOU DONE TODAY AND HOW DID YOU FEEL WHILE DOING IT?

WHAT WENT WELL DURING YOUR FAST TODAY?

IS THERE ANYTHING YOU'D DO DIFFERENTLY?

RECORD YOUR SUGAR VALUES

UPON WAKING

MIDDAY

BEFORE BED

HOW MANY HOURS DID YOU SLEEP? ◯

CIRCLE THE NUMBER THAT BEST DESCRIBES THE QUALITY OF YOUR SLEEP

1   2   3   4   5

Very Low   Low   Neutral   High   Very High

CIRCLE THE NUMBER THAT BEST DESCRIBES YOUR ENERGY LEVEL

1   2   3   4   5

Very Low   Low   Neutral   High   Very High

BREAKING YOUR FAST
WHEN DO YOU PLAN TO BREAK YOUR FAST?

HOW DO YOU PLAN TO BREAK YOUR FAST?

HOW DID YOU FEEL AFTER YOU BROKE YOUR FAST?

● ● ●

REFLECTION QUESTIONS

Please refer to the Questions section and select an area (or two) that resonates with you. Then choose and answer a question from the area or areas that most align with your thoughts and experiences today.

AREA OF FOCUS	MENTAL	EMOTIONAL	SPIRITUAL	PHYSICAL

QUESTION

ANSWER

● ● ●

FAST TRACKING

WHAT KIND OF FAST ARE YOU DOING?

IF YOUR FAST IS LONGER THAN ONE DAY, WHAT DAY OF YOUR FAST ARE YOU ON?

1   2   3   4   5

KETONE LEVEL
UPON WAKING

WHAT DAY ARE YOU ON IN YOUR MENSTRUAL CYCLE?

CIRCLE THE NUMBER THAT BEST DESCRIBES HOW YOU FELT AT THE END OF TODAY'S FAST

1	2	3	4	5
Angry	Sad	Neutral	Happy	Overjoyed

WHAT EXERCISE/ACTIVITY HAVE YOU DONE TODAY AND HOW DID YOU FEEL WHILE DOING IT?

WHAT WENT WELL DURING YOUR FAST TODAY?

IS THERE ANYTHING YOU'D DO DIFFERENTLY?

RECORD YOUR SUGAR VALUES

UPON WAKING

MIDDAY

BEFORE BED

HOW MANY HOURS DID YOU SLEEP?

CIRCLE THE NUMBER THAT BEST DESCRIBES THE QUALITY OF YOUR SLEEP

1	2	3	4	5
Very Low	Low	Neutral	High	Very High

CIRCLE THE NUMBER THAT BEST DESCRIBES YOUR ENERGY LEVEL

1	2	3	4	5
Very Low	Low	Neutral	High	Very High

BREAKING YOUR FAST
WHEN DO YOU PLAN TO BREAK YOUR FAST?

HOW DO YOU PLAN TO BREAK YOUR FAST?

HOW DID YOU FEEL AFTER YOU BROKE YOUR FAST?

• • •

REFLECTION QUESTIONS

Please refer to the Questions section and select an area (or two) that resonates with you. Then choose and answer a question from the area or areas that most align with your thoughts and experiences today.

AREA OF FOCUS	MENTAL	EMOTIONAL	SPIRITUAL	PHYSICAL

QUESTION

ANSWER

FAST TRACKING

WHAT KIND OF FAST ARE YOU DOING?

IF YOUR FAST IS LONGER THAN ONE DAY, WHAT DAY OF YOUR FAST ARE YOU ON?

1   2   3   4   5

KETONE LEVEL
UPON WAKING

WHAT DAY ARE YOU ON IN YOUR MENSTRUAL CYCLE?

CIRCLE THE NUMBER THAT BEST DESCRIBES HOW YOU FELT AT THE END OF TODAY'S FAST

1   2   3   4   5

Angry   Sad   Neutral   Happy   Overjoyed

WHAT EXERCISE/ACTIVITY HAVE YOU DONE TODAY AND HOW DID YOU FEEL WHILE DOING IT?

WHAT WENT WELL DURING YOUR FAST TODAY?

IS THERE ANYTHING YOU'D DO DIFFERENTLY?

RECORD YOUR SUGAR VALUES

UPON WAKING

MIDDAY

BEFORE BED

HOW MANY HOURS DID YOU SLEEP?

CIRCLE THE NUMBER THAT BEST DESCRIBES THE QUALITY OF YOUR SLEEP

1   2   3   4   5

Very Low   Low   Neutral   High   Very High

CIRCLE THE NUMBER THAT BEST DESCRIBES YOUR ENERGY LEVEL

1   2   3   4   5

Very Low   Low   Neutral   High   Very High

BREAKING YOUR FAST

WHEN DO YOU PLAN TO BREAK YOUR FAST?

HOW DO YOU PLAN TO BREAK YOUR FAST?

HOW DID YOU FEEL AFTER YOU BROKE YOUR FAST?

REFLECTION QUESTIONS

Please refer to the Questions section and select an area (or two) that resonates with you. Then choose and answer a question from the area or areas that most align with your thoughts and experiences today.

AREA OF FOCUS	MENTAL	EMOTIONAL	SPIRITUAL	PHYSICAL

QUESTION

ANSWER

FAST TRACKING

DATE ○ ○ ○

WHAT KIND OF FAST ARE YOU DOING?

IF YOUR FAST IS LONGER THAN ONE DAY, WHAT DAY OF YOUR FAST ARE YOU ON?

(1) (2) (3) (4) (5)

KETONE LEVEL
UPON WAKING

WHAT DAY ARE YOU ON IN YOUR MENSTRUAL CYCLE?

CIRCLE THE NUMBER THAT BEST DESCRIBES HOW YOU FELT AT THE END OF TODAY'S FAST

(1) (2) (3) (4) (5)
Angry   Sad   Neutral   Happy   Overjoyed

WHAT EXERCISE/ACTIVITY HAVE YOU DONE TODAY AND HOW DID YOU FEEL WHILE DOING IT?

WHAT WENT WELL DURING YOUR FAST TODAY?

IS THERE ANYTHING YOU'D DO DIFFERENTLY?

RECORD YOUR SUGAR VALUES

UPON WAKING

MIDDAY

BEFORE BED

HOW MANY HOURS DID YOU SLEEP?

CIRCLE THE NUMBER THAT BEST DESCRIBES THE QUALITY OF YOUR SLEEP

(1) (2) (3) (4) (5)
Very Low   Low   Neutral   High   Very High

CIRCLE THE NUMBER THAT BEST DESCRIBES YOUR ENERGY LEVEL

(1) (2) (3) (4) (5)
Very Low   Low   Neutral   High   Very High

BREAKING YOUR FAST
WHEN DO YOU PLAN TO BREAK YOUR FAST?

HOW DO YOU PLAN TO BREAK YOUR FAST?

HOW DID YOU FEEL AFTER YOU BROKE YOUR FAST?

REFLECTION QUESTIONS

Please refer to the Questions section and select an area (or two) that resonates with you. Then choose and answer a question from the area or areas that most align with your thoughts and experiences today.

AREA OF FOCUS	MENTAL	EMOTIONAL	SPIRITUAL	PHYSICAL

QUESTION

ANSWER

FAST TRACKING

WHAT KIND OF FAST ARE YOU DOING?

IF YOUR FAST IS LONGER THAN ONE DAY, WHAT DAY OF YOUR FAST ARE YOU ON?

1   2   3   4   5

KETONE LEVEL
UPON WAKING

WHAT DAY ARE YOU ON IN YOUR MENSTRUAL CYCLE?

CIRCLE THE NUMBER THAT BEST DESCRIBES HOW YOU FELT AT THE END OF TODAY'S FAST

1	2	3	4	5
Angry	Sad	Neutral	Happy	Overjoyed

WHAT EXERCISE/ACTIVITY HAVE YOU DONE TODAY AND HOW DID YOU FEEL WHILE DOING IT?

WHAT WENT WELL DURING YOUR FAST TODAY?

IS THERE ANYTHING YOU'D DO DIFFERENTLY?

RECORD YOUR SUGAR VALUES

UPON WAKING

MIDDAY

BEFORE BED

HOW MANY HOURS DID YOU SLEEP?

CIRCLE THE NUMBER THAT BEST DESCRIBES THE QUALITY OF YOUR SLEEP

1	2	3	4	5
Very Low	Low	Neutral	High	Very High

CIRCLE THE NUMBER THAT BEST DESCRIBES YOUR ENERGY LEVEL

1	2	3	4	5
Very Low	Low	Neutral	High	Very High

BREAKING YOUR FAST
WHEN DO YOU PLAN TO BREAK YOUR FAST?

HOW DO YOU PLAN TO BREAK YOUR FAST?

HOW DID YOU FEEL AFTER YOU BROKE YOUR FAST?

REFLECTION QUESTIONS

Please refer to the Questions section and select an area (or two) that resonates with you. Then choose and answer a question from the area or areas that most align with your thoughts and experiences today.

AREA OF FOCUS	MENTAL	EMOTIONAL	SPIRITUAL	PHYSICAL

QUESTION

ANSWER

" —

Fasting isn't about eating fewer calories or starving yourself. It's about honoring your body's ability to heal in the absence of food and in the presence of food.

"

You don't need
motivation,
you need
momentum.

FAST TRACKING

WHAT KIND OF FAST ARE YOU DOING?

IF YOUR FAST IS LONGER THAN ONE DAY, WHAT DAY OF YOUR FAST ARE YOU ON?

1   2   3   4   5

KETONE LEVEL
UPON WAKING

WHAT DAY ARE YOU ON IN YOUR MENSTRUAL CYCLE?

CIRCLE THE NUMBER THAT BEST DESCRIBES HOW YOU FELT AT THE END OF TODAY'S FAST

1   2   3   4   5

Angry   Sad   Neutral   Happy   Overjoyed

WHAT EXERCISE/ACTIVITY HAVE YOU DONE TODAY AND HOW DID YOU FEEL WHILE DOING IT?

WHAT WENT WELL DURING YOUR FAST TODAY?

IS THERE ANYTHING YOU'D DO DIFFERENTLY?

RECORD YOUR SUGAR VALUES

UPON WAKING

MIDDAY

BEFORE BED

HOW MANY HOURS DID YOU SLEEP?

CIRCLE THE NUMBER THAT BEST DESCRIBES THE QUALITY OF YOUR SLEEP

1   2   3   4   5

Very Low   Low   Neutral   High   Very High

CIRCLE THE NUMBER THAT BEST DESCRIBES YOUR ENERGY LEVEL

1   2   3   4   5

Very Low   Low   Neutral   High   Very High

BREAKING YOUR FAST
WHEN DO YOU PLAN TO BREAK YOUR FAST?

HOW DO YOU PLAN TO BREAK YOUR FAST?

HOW DID YOU FEEL AFTER YOU BROKE YOUR FAST?

REFLECTION QUESTIONS

Please refer to the Questions section and select an area (or two) that resonates with you. Then choose and answer a question from the area or areas that most align with your thoughts and experiences today.

AREA OF FOCUS	MENTAL	EMOTIONAL	SPIRITUAL	PHYSICAL

QUESTION

ANSWER

FAST TRACKING

WHAT KIND OF FAST ARE YOU DOING?

IF YOUR FAST IS LONGER THAN ONE DAY, WHAT DAY OF YOUR FAST ARE YOU ON?

1   2   3   4   5

KETONE LEVEL
UPON WAKING

WHAT DAY ARE YOU ON IN YOUR MENSTRUAL CYCLE?

CIRCLE THE NUMBER THAT BEST DESCRIBES HOW YOU FELT AT THE END OF TODAY'S FAST

1   2   3   4   5
Angry   Sad   Neutral   Happy   Overjoyed

WHAT EXERCISE/ACTIVITY HAVE YOU DONE TODAY AND HOW DID YOU FEEL WHILE DOING IT?

WHAT WENT WELL DURING YOUR FAST TODAY?

IS THERE ANYTHING YOU'D DO DIFFERENTLY?

RECORD YOUR SUGAR VALUES

UPON WAKING

MIDDAY

BEFORE BED

HOW MANY HOURS DID YOU SLEEP?

CIRCLE THE NUMBER THAT BEST DESCRIBES THE QUALITY OF YOUR SLEEP

1   2   3   4   5
Very Low   Low   Neutral   High   Very High

CIRCLE THE NUMBER THAT BEST DESCRIBES YOUR ENERGY LEVEL

1   2   3   4   5
Very Low   Low   Neutral   High   Very High

BREAKING YOUR FAST

WHEN DO YOU PLAN TO BREAK YOUR FAST?

HOW DO YOU PLAN TO BREAK YOUR FAST?

HOW DID YOU FEEL AFTER YOU BROKE YOUR FAST?

REFLECTION QUESTIONS

Please refer to the Questions section and select an area (or two) that resonates with you. Then choose and answer a question from the area or areas that most align with your thoughts and experiences today.

| AREA OF FOCUS | MENTAL | EMOTIONAL | SPIRITUAL | PHYSICAL |

QUESTION

ANSWER

FAST TRACKING

DATE ◯ ◯ ◯

WHAT KIND OF FAST ARE YOU DOING?

IF YOUR FAST IS LONGER THAN ONE DAY, WHAT DAY OF YOUR FAST ARE YOU ON?

1   2   3   4   5

KETONE LEVEL
UPON WAKING

WHAT DAY ARE YOU ON IN YOUR MENSTRUAL CYCLE?

CIRCLE THE NUMBER THAT BEST DESCRIBES HOW YOU FELT AT THE END OF TODAY'S FAST

1   2   3   4   5

Angry   Sad   Neutral   Happy   Overjoyed

WHAT EXERCISE/ACTIVITY HAVE YOU DONE TODAY AND HOW DID YOU FEEL WHILE DOING IT?

WHAT WENT WELL DURING YOUR FAST TODAY?

IS THERE ANYTHING YOU'D DO DIFFERENTLY?

RECORD YOUR SUGAR VALUES

UPON WAKING

MIDDAY

BEFORE BED

HOW MANY HOURS DID YOU SLEEP? ◯

CIRCLE THE NUMBER THAT BEST DESCRIBES THE QUALITY OF YOUR SLEEP

1   2   3   4   5

Very Low   Low   Neutral   High   Very High

CIRCLE THE NUMBER THAT BEST DESCRIBES YOUR ENERGY LEVEL

1   2   3   4   5

Very Low   Low   Neutral   High   Very High

BREAKING YOUR FAST

WHEN DO YOU PLAN TO BREAK YOUR FAST?

HOW DO YOU PLAN TO BREAK YOUR FAST?

HOW DID YOU FEEL AFTER YOU BROKE YOUR FAST?

●●●

REFLECTION QUESTIONS

Please refer to the Questions section and select an area (or two) that resonates with you. Then choose and answer a question from the area or areas that most align with your thoughts and experiences today.

AREA OF FOCUS	MENTAL	EMOTIONAL	SPIRITUAL	PHYSICAL

QUESTION

ANSWER

● ● ●

FAST TRACKING

DATE ◯ ◯ ◯

WHAT KIND OF FAST ARE YOU DOING?

IF YOUR FAST IS LONGER THAN ONE DAY, WHAT DAY OF YOUR FAST ARE YOU ON?

(1) (2) (3) (4) (5)

KETONE LEVEL
UPON WAKING

WHAT DAY ARE YOU ON IN YOUR MENSTRUAL CYCLE?

CIRCLE THE NUMBER THAT BEST DESCRIBES HOW YOU FELT AT THE END OF TODAY'S FAST

(1) (2) (3) (4) (5)

Angry   Sad   Neutral   Happy   Overjoyed

WHAT EXERCISE/ACTIVITY HAVE YOU DONE TODAY AND HOW DID YOU FEEL WHILE DOING IT?

WHAT WENT WELL DURING YOUR FAST TODAY?

IS THERE ANYTHING YOU'D DO DIFFERENTLY?

RECORD YOUR SUGAR VALUES

UPON WAKING

MIDDAY

BEFORE BED

HOW MANY HOURS DID YOU SLEEP?

CIRCLE THE NUMBER THAT BEST DESCRIBES THE QUALITY OF YOUR SLEEP

(1) (2) (3) (4) (5)

Very Low   Low   Neutral   High   Very High

CIRCLE THE NUMBER THAT BEST DESCRIBES YOUR ENERGY LEVEL

(1) (2) (3) (4) (5)

Very Low   Low   Neutral   High   Very High

BREAKING YOUR FAST
WHEN DO YOU PLAN TO BREAK YOUR FAST?

HOW DO YOU PLAN TO BREAK YOUR FAST?

HOW DID YOU FEEL AFTER YOU BROKE YOUR FAST?

● ● ●

REFLECTION QUESTIONS

Please refer to the Questions section and select an area (or two) that resonates with you. Then choose and answer a question from the area or areas that most align with your thoughts and experiences today.

| AREA OF FOCUS | MENTAL | EMOTIONAL | SPIRITUAL | PHYSICAL |

QUESTION

ANSWER

FAST TRACKING

DATE ◯ ◯ ◯

WHAT KIND OF FAST ARE YOU DOING?

IF YOUR FAST IS LONGER THAN ONE DAY, WHAT DAY OF YOUR FAST ARE YOU ON?

(1) (2) (3) (4) (5)

KETONE LEVEL
UPON WAKING

WHAT DAY ARE YOU ON IN YOUR MENSTRUAL CYCLE?

CIRCLE THE NUMBER THAT BEST DESCRIBES HOW YOU FELT AT THE END OF TODAY'S FAST

(1) (2) (3) (4) (5)

Angry   Sad   Neutral   Happy   Overjoyed

WHAT EXERCISE/ACTIVITY HAVE YOU DONE TODAY AND HOW DID YOU FEEL WHILE DOING IT?

WHAT WENT WELL DURING YOUR FAST TODAY?

IS THERE ANYTHING YOU'D DO DIFFERENTLY?

RECORD YOUR SUGAR VALUES

UPON WAKING

MIDDAY

BEFORE BED

HOW MANY HOURS DID YOU SLEEP? ◯

CIRCLE THE NUMBER THAT BEST DESCRIBES THE QUALITY OF YOUR SLEEP

(1) (2) (3) (4) (5)

Very Low   Low   Neutral   High   Very High

CIRCLE THE NUMBER THAT BEST DESCRIBES YOUR ENERGY LEVEL

(1) (2) (3) (4) (5)

Very Low   Low   Neutral   High   Very High

BREAKING YOUR FAST

WHEN DO YOU PLAN TO BREAK YOUR FAST?

HOW DO YOU PLAN TO BREAK YOUR FAST?

HOW DID YOU FEEL AFTER YOU BROKE YOUR FAST?

● ● ●

REFLECTION QUESTIONS

Please refer to the Questions section and select an area (or two) that resonates with you. Then choose and answer a question from the area or areas that most align with your thoughts and experiences today.

AREA OF FOCUS	MENTAL	EMOTIONAL	SPIRITUAL	PHYSICAL

QUESTION

ANSWER

FAST TRACKING

DATE ⬤ ⬤ ⬤

WHAT KIND OF FAST ARE YOU DOING?

IF YOUR FAST IS LONGER THAN ONE DAY, WHAT DAY OF YOUR FAST ARE YOU ON?

1   2   3   4   5

KETONE LEVEL
UPON WAKING

WHAT DAY ARE YOU ON IN YOUR MENSTRUAL CYCLE?

CIRCLE THE NUMBER THAT BEST DESCRIBES HOW YOU FELT AT THE END OF TODAY'S FAST

1   2   3   4   5

Angry   Sad   Neutral   Happy   Overjoyed

WHAT EXERCISE/ACTIVITY HAVE YOU DONE TODAY AND HOW DID YOU FEEL WHILE DOING IT?

WHAT WENT WELL DURING YOUR FAST TODAY?

IS THERE ANYTHING YOU'D DO DIFFERENTLY?

RECORD YOUR SUGAR VALUES

UPON WAKING

MIDDAY

BEFORE BED

HOW MANY HOURS DID YOU SLEEP?

CIRCLE THE NUMBER THAT BEST DESCRIBES THE QUALITY OF YOUR SLEEP

1   2   3   4   5

Very Low   Low   Neutral   High   Very High

CIRCLE THE NUMBER THAT BEST DESCRIBES YOUR ENERGY LEVEL

1   2   3   4   5

Very Low   Low   Neutral   High   Very High

BREAKING YOUR FAST

WHEN DO YOU PLAN TO BREAK YOUR FAST?

HOW DO YOU PLAN TO BREAK YOUR FAST?

HOW DID YOU FEEL AFTER YOU BROKE YOUR FAST?

REFLECTION QUESTIONS

Please refer to the Questions section and select an area (or two) that resonates with you. Then choose and answer a question from the area or areas that most align with your thoughts and experiences today.

| AREA OF FOCUS | MENTAL | EMOTIONAL | SPIRITUAL | PHYSICAL |

QUESTION

ANSWER

"

Your body is
listening to
everything your
mind is saying.

"

If you start fasting
today, your
immune system
will be stronger
by tomorrow.

FAST TRACKING

WHAT KIND OF FAST ARE YOU DOING?

IF YOUR FAST IS LONGER THAN ONE DAY, WHAT DAY OF YOUR FAST ARE YOU ON?

1   2   3   4   5

KETONE LEVEL
UPON WAKING

WHAT DAY ARE YOU ON IN YOUR MENSTRUAL CYCLE?

CIRCLE THE NUMBER THAT BEST DESCRIBES HOW YOU FELT AT THE END OF TODAY'S FAST

1	2	3	4	5
Angry	Sad	Neutral	Happy	Overjoyed

WHAT EXERCISE/ACTIVITY HAVE YOU DONE TODAY AND HOW DID YOU FEEL WHILE DOING IT?

WHAT WENT WELL DURING YOUR FAST TODAY?

IS THERE ANYTHING YOU'D DO DIFFERENTLY?

RECORD YOUR SUGAR VALUES

UPON WAKING

MIDDAY

BEFORE BED

HOW MANY HOURS DID YOU SLEEP?

CIRCLE THE NUMBER THAT BEST DESCRIBES THE QUALITY OF YOUR SLEEP

1	2	3	4	5
Very Low	Low	Neutral	High	Very High

CIRCLE THE NUMBER THAT BEST DESCRIBES YOUR ENERGY LEVEL

1	2	3	4	5
Very Low	Low	Neutral	High	Very High

BREAKING YOUR FAST
WHEN DO YOU PLAN TO BREAK YOUR FAST?

HOW DO YOU PLAN TO BREAK YOUR FAST?

HOW DID YOU FEEL AFTER YOU BROKE YOUR FAST?

REFLECTION QUESTIONS

Please refer to the Questions section and select an area (or two) that resonates with you. Then choose and answer a question from the area or areas that most align with your thoughts and experiences today.

AREA OF FOCUS	MENTAL	EMOTIONAL	SPIRITUAL	PHYSICAL

QUESTION

ANSWER

FAST TRACKING

WHAT KIND OF FAST ARE YOU DOING?

IF YOUR FAST IS LONGER THAN ONE DAY, WHAT DAY OF YOUR FAST ARE YOU ON?

(1)　(2)　(3)　(4)　(5)

KETONE LEVEL
UPON WAKING

WHAT DAY ARE YOU ON IN YOUR MENSTRUAL CYCLE?

CIRCLE THE NUMBER THAT BEST DESCRIBES HOW YOU FELT AT THE END OF TODAY'S FAST

(1)　(2)　(3)　(4)　(5)

Angry　Sad　Neutral　Happy　Overjoyed

WHAT EXERCISE/ACTIVITY HAVE YOU DONE TODAY AND HOW DID YOU FEEL WHILE DOING IT?

WHAT WENT WELL DURING YOUR FAST TODAY?

IS THERE ANYTHING YOU'D DO DIFFERENTLY?

RECORD YOUR SUGAR VALUES

UPON WAKING

MIDDAY

BEFORE BED

HOW MANY HOURS DID YOU SLEEP?

CIRCLE THE NUMBER THAT BEST DESCRIBES THE QUALITY OF YOUR SLEEP

(1)　(2)　(3)　(4)　(5)

Very Low　Low　Neutral　High　Very High

CIRCLE THE NUMBER THAT BEST DESCRIBES YOUR ENERGY LEVEL

(1)　(2)　(3)　(4)　(5)

Very Low　Low　Neutral　High　Very High

BREAKING YOUR FAST
WHEN DO YOU PLAN TO BREAK YOUR FAST?

HOW DO YOU PLAN TO BREAK YOUR FAST?

HOW DID YOU FEEL AFTER YOU BROKE YOUR FAST?

REFLECTION QUESTIONS

Please refer to the Questions section and select an area (or two) that resonates with you. Then choose and answer a question from the area or areas that most align with your thoughts and experiences today.

AREA OF FOCUS	MENTAL	EMOTIONAL	SPIRITUAL	PHYSICAL

QUESTION

ANSWER

FAST TRACKING

WHAT KIND OF FAST ARE YOU DOING?

IF YOUR FAST IS LONGER THAN ONE DAY, WHAT DAY OF YOUR FAST ARE YOU ON?

1   2   3   4   5

KETONE LEVEL
UPON WAKING

WHAT DAY ARE YOU ON IN YOUR MENSTRUAL CYCLE?

CIRCLE THE NUMBER THAT BEST DESCRIBES HOW YOU FELT AT THE END OF TODAY'S FAST

1	2	3	4	5
Angry	Sad	Neutral	Happy	Overjoyed

WHAT EXERCISE/ACTIVITY HAVE YOU DONE TODAY AND HOW DID YOU FEEL WHILE DOING IT?

WHAT WENT WELL DURING YOUR FAST TODAY?

IS THERE ANYTHING YOU'D DO DIFFERENTLY?

RECORD YOUR SUGAR VALUES

UPON WAKING

MIDDAY

BEFORE BED

HOW MANY HOURS DID YOU SLEEP?

CIRCLE THE NUMBER THAT BEST DESCRIBES THE QUALITY OF YOUR SLEEP

1	2	3	4	5
Very Low	Low	Neutral	High	Very High

CIRCLE THE NUMBER THAT BEST DESCRIBES YOUR ENERGY LEVEL

1	2	3	4	5
Very Low	Low	Neutral	High	Very High

BREAKING YOUR FAST
WHEN DO YOU PLAN TO BREAK YOUR FAST?

HOW DO YOU PLAN TO BREAK YOUR FAST?

HOW DID YOU FEEL AFTER YOU BROKE YOUR FAST?

REFLECTION QUESTIONS

Please refer to the Questions section and select an area (or two) that resonates with you. Then choose and answer a question from the area or areas that most align with your thoughts and experiences today.

AREA OF FOCUS	MENTAL	EMOTIONAL	SPIRITUAL	PHYSICAL

QUESTION

ANSWER

FAST TRACKING

WHAT KIND OF FAST ARE YOU DOING?

IF YOUR FAST IS LONGER THAN ONE DAY, WHAT DAY OF YOUR FAST ARE YOU ON?

1   2   3   4   5

KETONE LEVEL
UPON WAKING

WHAT DAY ARE YOU ON IN YOUR MENSTRUAL CYCLE?

CIRCLE THE NUMBER THAT BEST DESCRIBES HOW YOU FELT AT THE END OF TODAY'S FAST

1	2	3	4	5
Angry	Sad	Neutral	Happy	Overjoyed

WHAT EXERCISE/ACTIVITY HAVE YOU DONE TODAY AND HOW DID YOU FEEL WHILE DOING IT?

WHAT WENT WELL DURING YOUR FAST TODAY?

IS THERE ANYTHING YOU'D DO DIFFERENTLY?

RECORD YOUR SUGAR VALUES

UPON WAKING

MIDDAY

BEFORE BED

HOW MANY HOURS DID YOU SLEEP?

CIRCLE THE NUMBER THAT BEST DESCRIBES THE QUALITY OF YOUR SLEEP

1	2	3	4	5
Very Low	Low	Neutral	High	Very High

CIRCLE THE NUMBER THAT BEST DESCRIBES YOUR ENERGY LEVEL

1	2	3	4	5
Very Low	Low	Neutral	High	Very High

BREAKING YOUR FAST
WHEN DO YOU PLAN TO BREAK YOUR FAST?

HOW DO YOU PLAN TO BREAK YOUR FAST?

HOW DID YOU FEEL AFTER YOU BROKE YOUR FAST?

REFLECTION QUESTIONS

Please refer to the Questions section and select an area (or two) that resonates with you. Then choose and answer a question from the area or areas that most align with your thoughts and experiences today.

AREA OF FOCUS	MENTAL	EMOTIONAL	SPIRITUAL	PHYSICAL

QUESTION

ANSWER

FAST TRACKING

WHAT KIND OF FAST ARE YOU DOING?

IF YOUR FAST IS LONGER THAN ONE DAY, WHAT DAY OF YOUR FAST ARE YOU ON?

1   2   3   4   5

KETONE LEVEL
UPON WAKING

WHAT DAY ARE YOU ON IN YOUR MENSTRUAL CYCLE?

CIRCLE THE NUMBER THAT BEST DESCRIBES HOW YOU FELT AT THE END OF TODAY'S FAST

1   2   3   4   5

Angry   Sad   Neutral   Happy   Overjoyed

WHAT EXERCISE/ACTIVITY HAVE YOU DONE TODAY AND HOW DID YOU FEEL WHILE DOING IT?

WHAT WENT WELL DURING YOUR FAST TODAY?

IS THERE ANYTHING YOU'D DO DIFFERENTLY?

RECORD YOUR SUGAR VALUES

UPON WAKING

MIDDAY

BEFORE BED

HOW MANY HOURS DID YOU SLEEP?

CIRCLE THE NUMBER THAT BEST DESCRIBES THE QUALITY OF YOUR SLEEP

1   2   3   4   5

Very Low   Low   Neutral   High   Very High

CIRCLE THE NUMBER THAT BEST DESCRIBES YOUR ENERGY LEVEL

1   2   3   4   5

Very Low   Low   Neutral   High   Very High

BREAKING YOUR FAST
WHEN DO YOU PLAN TO BREAK YOUR FAST?

HOW DO YOU PLAN TO BREAK YOUR FAST?

HOW DID YOU FEEL AFTER YOU BROKE YOUR FAST?

REFLECTION QUESTIONS

Please refer to the Questions section and select an area (or two) that resonates with you. Then choose and answer a question from the area or areas that most align with your thoughts and experiences today.

AREA OF FOCUS	MENTAL	EMOTIONAL	SPIRITUAL	PHYSICAL

QUESTION

ANSWER

FAST TRACKING

WHAT KIND OF FAST ARE YOU DOING?

IF YOUR FAST IS LONGER THAN ONE DAY, WHAT DAY OF YOUR FAST ARE YOU ON?

1   2   3   4   5

KETONE LEVEL
UPON WAKING

WHAT DAY ARE YOU ON IN YOUR MENSTRUAL CYCLE?

CIRCLE THE NUMBER THAT BEST DESCRIBES HOW YOU FELT AT THE END OF TODAY'S FAST

1	2	3	4	5
Angry	Sad	Neutral	Happy	Overjoyed

WHAT EXERCISE/ACTIVITY HAVE YOU DONE TODAY AND HOW DID YOU FEEL WHILE DOING IT?

WHAT WENT WELL DURING YOUR FAST TODAY?

IS THERE ANYTHING YOU'D DO DIFFERENTLY?

RECORD YOUR SUGAR VALUES

UPON WAKING

MIDDAY

BEFORE BED

HOW MANY HOURS DID YOU SLEEP?

CIRCLE THE NUMBER THAT BEST DESCRIBES THE QUALITY OF YOUR SLEEP

1	2	3	4	5
Very Low	Low	Neutral	High	Very High

CIRCLE THE NUMBER THAT BEST DESCRIBES YOUR ENERGY LEVEL

1	2	3	4	5
Very Low	Low	Neutral	High	Very High

BREAKING YOUR FAST
WHEN DO YOU PLAN TO BREAK YOUR FAST?

HOW DO YOU PLAN TO BREAK YOUR FAST?

HOW DID YOU FEEL AFTER YOU BROKE YOUR FAST?

REFLECTION QUESTIONS

Please refer to the Questions section and select an area (or two) that resonates with you. Then choose and answer a question from the area or areas that most align with your thoughts and experiences today.

AREA OF FOCUS	MENTAL	EMOTIONAL	SPIRITUAL	PHYSICAL

QUESTION

ANSWER

Fasting heals and so does food.

"

Your body was born with an innate intelligence. It wants to heal, and fasting allows it to do exactly that.

PART IV

Activity Pages

Fasting allows you to get to know your thoughts, beliefs, and behaviors from a new lens. Many people discover that not only do they have more time while fasting, but they also gain more clarity about their relationship to food, how they feel about their body, and what health habits they want to bring into their lives. To best assist you in that discovery process, I have included some activity pages that will help you sort out the beliefs that may be bubbling to the surface during your fast. The following are the pages I have included here for you and suggestions on how you can best use them.

COLORING PAGES

I Got This

Knowledge Is My Fuel

I Am Healing

My Body Is Powerful

If you haven't colored since you were a kid, now is the time! It's so relaxing. In fact, according to the Mayo Clinic not only does coloring calm the brain and help your body relax, but it can improve sleep while decreasing fatigue, body aches, heart rate, respiration, and depression and anxiety. All of this makes it a great activity to do when you are in a fasted state. If you find it hard to quiet your mind while you are fasting, just grab some colored pencils and doodle on these pages. You may be surprised at how quickly it calms you.

I MATTER

As women, too often we only see our flaws. Unfortunately, the patriarchal world we live in can sometimes make us feel like we are not enough. If you have ever felt unseen and unheard, please know that you matter! You have so many unique and wonderful gifts that you bring the world. So let's highlight those gifts and put them front of mind. Using the clarity that fasting offers you, take a moment to sit with this activity page and brag about yourself. What are your superpowers? Maybe you are kind, courageous, creative, strong, beautiful, caring, tenacious, or deeply wise. Put all these attributes into I am statements. Affirmations you can anchor to when you feel lost. For some of us, it can be hard to brag about ourselves. Yet, I want you to brag away. This is the type of exercise you don't want to overthink. Let these statements come from your heart. The first thoughts that come to your mind

●●●

are often the most accurate ones. I like to do this exercise as I sip a cup of my favorite tea in a quiet, soothing place in my home while listening to music that opens my heart. If you allow it, this can be one of the most empowering activities in this journal. Enjoy!

MY CIRCLE OF SUPPORT

This exercise holds a special place in my heart—a lesson I learned years ago from one of my patients who was on a remarkable healing journey while battling metastatic breast cancer. Initially given only three months to live, she defied the odds and turned that prognosis into a full decade of life. During this time, she meticulously assessed every aspect of her life, including her relationships. In her kitchen, she displayed a picture representing her "circle of support." Those closest to the inner circle represented the positive influences in her life, individuals who truly supported her healing process. The outer circles, on the other hand, consisted of people with whom she needed to limit interactions, as they seemed to drain her of health and energy. She would pencil in people's names and arrange and rearrange them within the circles as she saw fit. This exercise helped to ensure that she surrounded herself with positive healing energy.

I've included this exercise here for you so that you can embark on a similar journey of self-reflection. As hard as it can be to accept, we could have individuals in our lives who, rather than supporting our healing, introduce toxicity and negativity. On the flip side, we're fortunate to have amazing cheerleaders who make the healing process joyful and effortless. This exercise will help you identify these individuals with clarity. Remember, relationships can evolve, so don't hesitate to rearrange people within the circles as your needs and circumstances change.

THE BEAUTY OF GRATITUDE

It's easy to get distracted by your problems. The human brain is wired to fix these problems which often leaves little time for us to focus on what we are grateful for. Typically, the mind will quiet the longer you fast. As the mind calms, the heart can often hear the voice of your heart start talking louder to you. Your heart's voice is full of gratitude. Let's capture its voice! The I am grateful activity page is to write down the words your heart speaks to you. When you go back to food and the business of your life you may lose your heart's voice. On days you feel like you've lost your way, come back to this

● ● ●

gratitude page. It will remind you of the important anchors in your life that bring you joy.

HEALTH GOALS

How many times have we set a health goal, only to lose our focus with that goal weeks later? A well-executed plan combined with a community of support is massively important when it comes to hitting your goals. You will get so much clarity when you are in the fasted state, making it a great time to set some clear health goals that you are guaranteed to hit! In this activity page, you will see that you can write your health goal in the center and then follow the prompts it gives you in the squares, flowers, and arrows that surround your goal. If your goal was a meal you were making, the prompts that surround the health goal bowl are the ingredients needed to succeed. I know you will find that this a super fun way to not only set your health goals, but it's a fabulous way to see how well-supported you are in making sure you achieve that goal.

KIND THINGS I WILL SAY TO MYSELF IN THE MIRROR

All too often we look in the mirror and see all the things we don't like about our bodies. We can be our harshest critic. Let's change that! The mirror exercise is for you to take a moment and reflect on all the kind things you want to tell your body. Write them down on this page and come back to this picture as often. All too often we want others to be kind to us, but don't take inventory of how kind we are to ourselves. When you are on a healing journey, your self-talk matters. Use this exercise to think of all the things you love about your body. Doesn't matter how big or small the statement is, it's a reminder to love yourself and this beautiful body you get to live in. You may even tear this page out of the journal and tape it to your mirror to remind you to be gentle and kind to yourself.

THINGS THAT MAKE ME BEAUTIFUL

As women, we can be so hard on ourselves. Our culture has told us we need to look, think, and act in a certain way. When we don't measure up to society's expectations, we start to turn on ourselves and say harsh things to ourselves. There are so many parts of you that make you beautiful. Parts that you may not recognize because you have been judging yourself against a society that has taught you what beauty is supposed to look like. With this activity page, you get to amplify all the unique parts of you that make you uniquely beautiful. Beauty doesn't have to be the size of clothes you fit into or the new outfit you bought. Beauty can be your humble heart, or vibrant energy, or maybe it's your brilliant mind. In this exercise I want you to count all the ways you are beautiful. Brag about yourself to yourself! That's what this exercise is for. Dip into the confidence that fills you that perhaps you would never articulate to anyone else. Let's bring all the parts that make you beautiful to the surface now.

WHAT I LOVE ABOUT MY BODY

It's easy to go into fix-it mode with your body. You want to lose weight, build more muscle, and slow down the aging process—great goals. But let's not lose sight of what is already brilliant about your body. Whether it's the color of your hair, or the ease with which your body moves, or perhaps you love the softness of your skin. No matter how small, let's point out here on this activity page all the ways your body is serving you well. The more you speak kindly to your body, the more it will respond by giving you a vibrant, healthy home to live in.

● ● ●

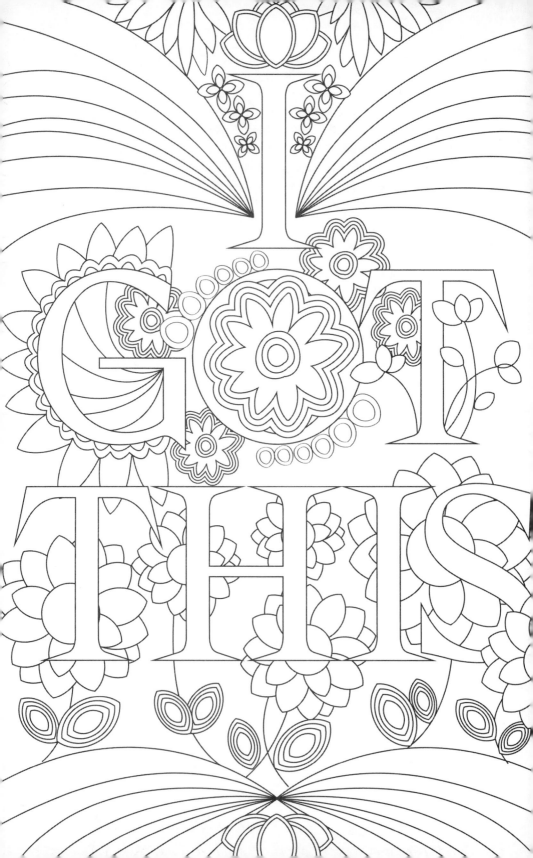

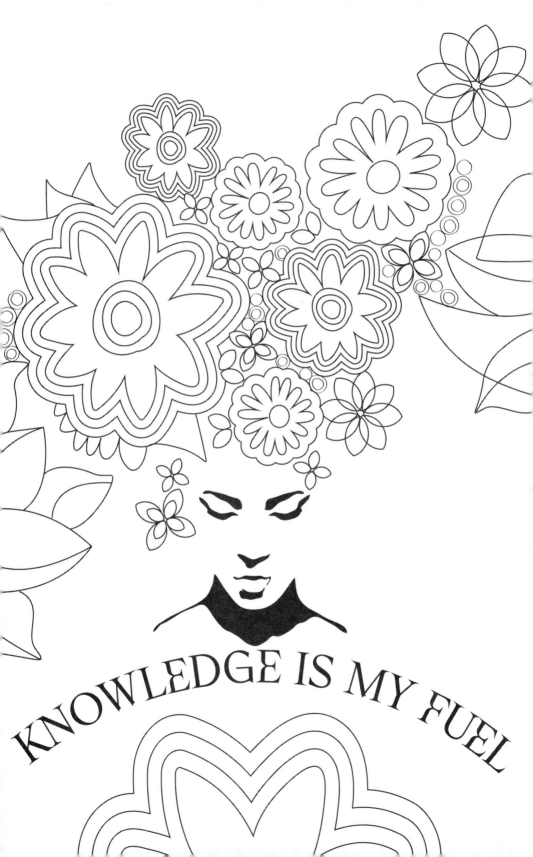

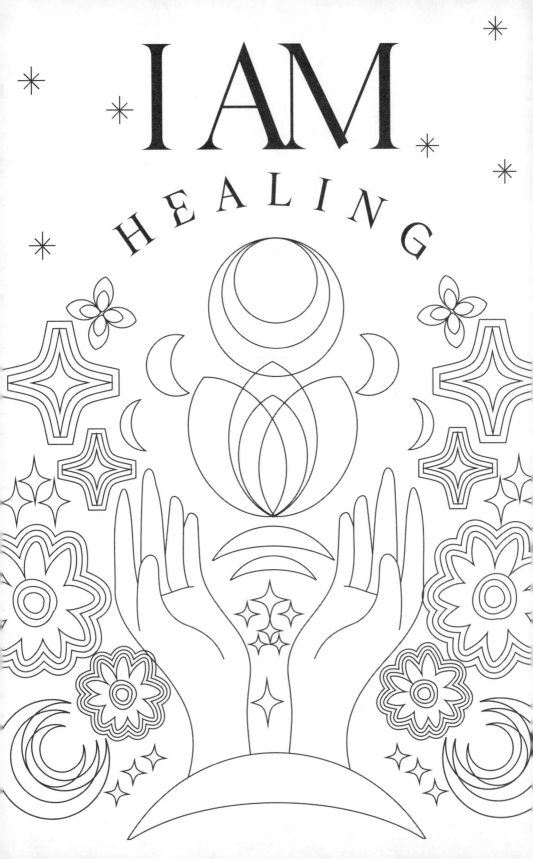

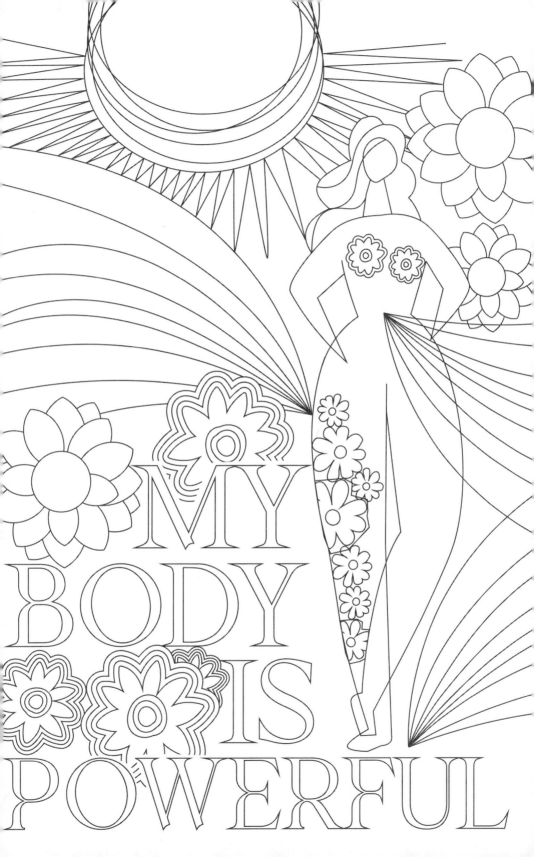

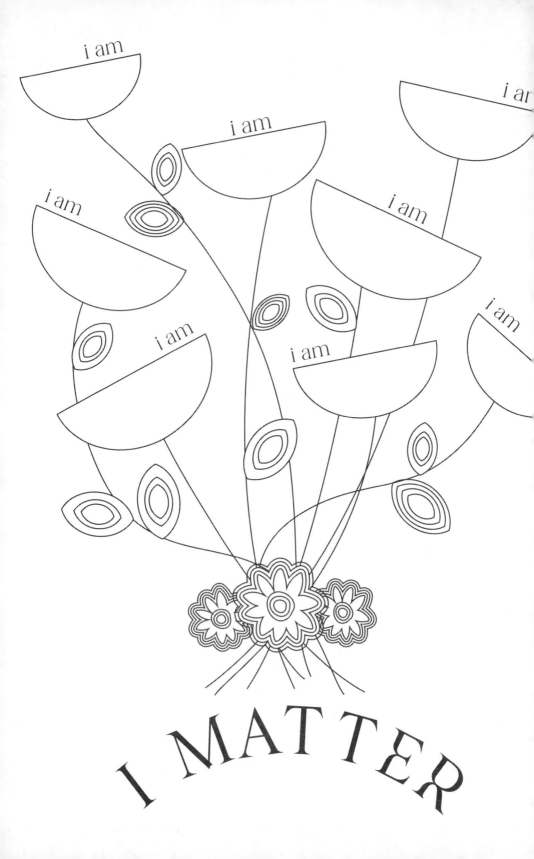

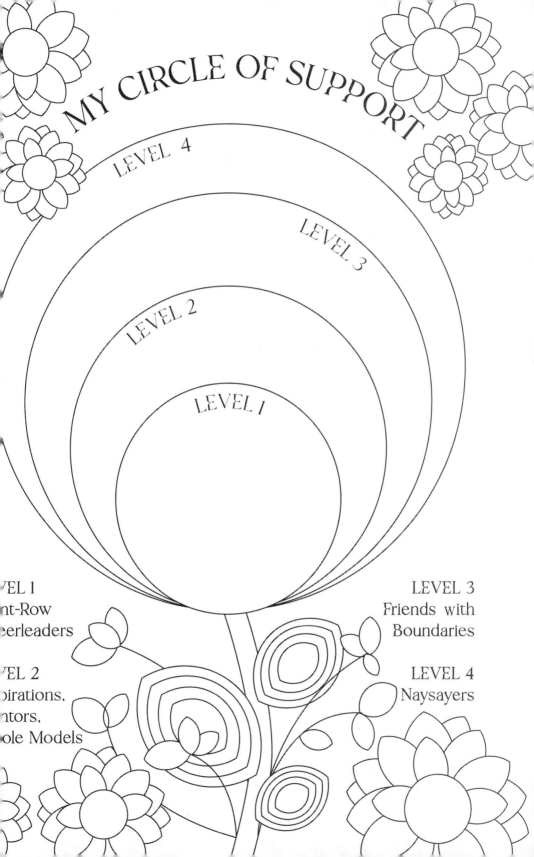

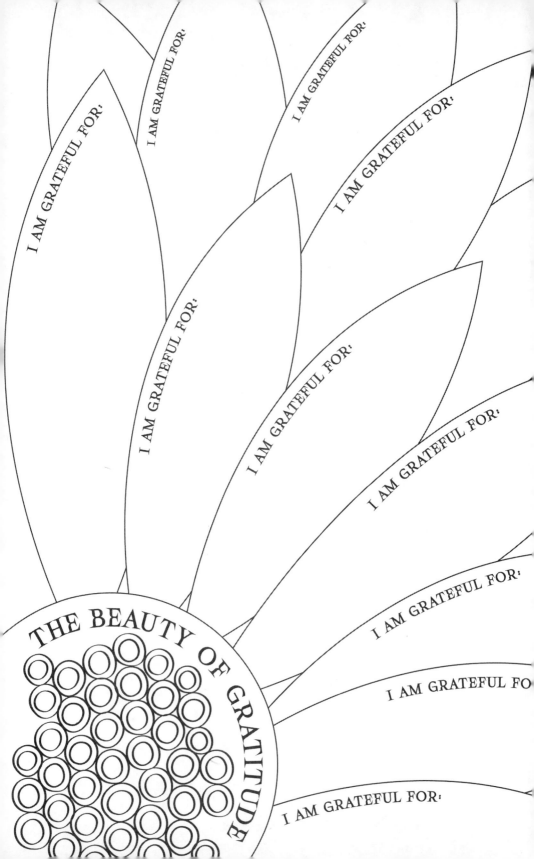

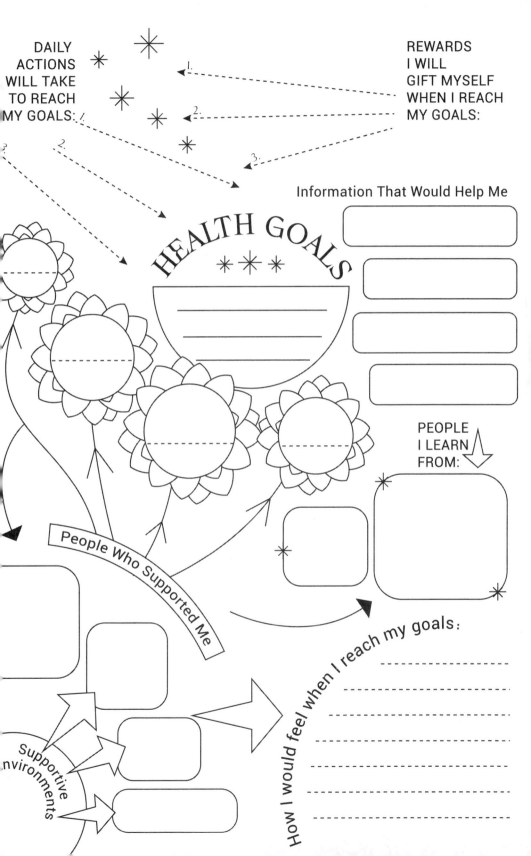

DAILY
ACTIONS
WILL TAKE
TO REACH
MY GOALS:

1.
2.
3.
2.

REWARDS
I WILL
GIFT MYSELF
WHEN I REACH
MY GOALS:

1.
2.
3.

Information That Would Help Me

HEALTH GOALS
✳✳✳

PEOPLE
I LEARN
FROM:

People Who Supported Me

How I would feel when I reach my goals:

Supportive Environments

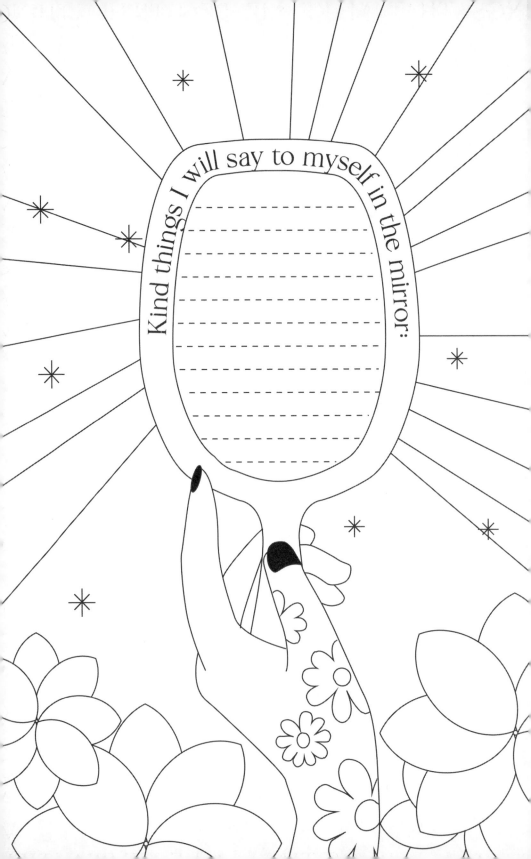

Kind things I will say to myself in the mirror:

THINGS THAT MAKE ME BEAUTIFUL. THINGS
THAT MAKE ME BEAUTIFUL. THINGS THAT
MAKE ME BEAUTIFUL. THINGS THAT MAKE M
BEAUTIFUL. THINGS THAT MAKE ME BEAUTIFUL
THINGS THAT MAKE ME BEAUTIFUL. THINGS
THAT MAKE ME BEAUTIFUL. THINGS THAT MAKE M
BEAUTIFUL. THINGS THAT MAKE ME BEAUTIFUL
THINGS THAT MAKE ME BEAUTIFUL. THINGS
THAT MAKE ME BEAUTIFUL. THINGS THAT MAKE M
BEAUTIFUL. THINGS THAT MAKE ME BEAUTIFUL
THINGS THAT MAKE ME BEAUTIFUL. THINGS
THAT MAKE ME BEAUTIFUL. THINGS THAT MAKE M
BEAUTIFUL. THINGS THAT MAKE ME BEAUTIFUL
THINGS THAT MAKE ME BEAUTIFUL. THINGS THA
THAT MAKE ME BEAUTIFUL. THINGS THAT MAKE M
BEAUTIFUL. THINGS THAT MAKE ME BEAUTIFU
THINGS THAT MAKE ME BEAUTIFUL. THINGS THA
THAT MAKE ME BEAUTIFUL. THINGS THAT MAKE M
BEAUTIFUL. THINGS THAT MAKE ME BEAUTIFUL
THINGS THAT MAKE ME BEAUTIFUL. THINGS THA
THAT MAKE ME BEAUTIFUL. THINGS THAT MAKE M
BEAUTIFUL. THINGS THAT MAKE ME BEAUTIFUL.

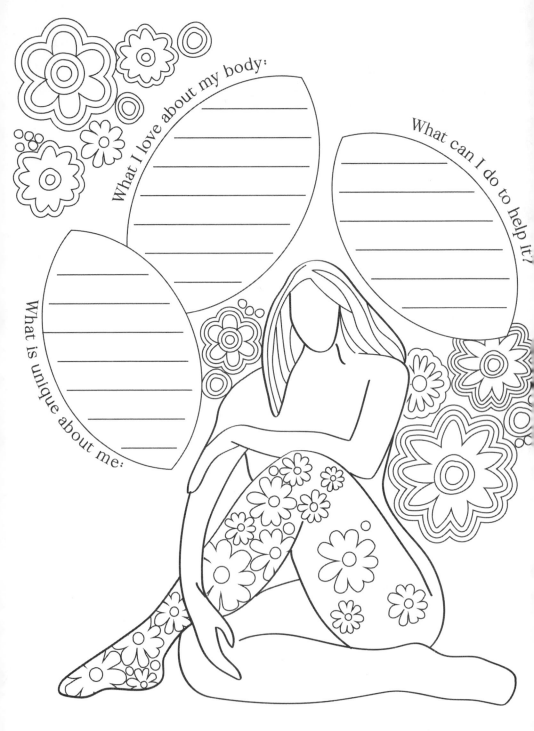

What I love about my body:

_____
_____
_____
_____
_____
_____

What can I do to help it?

_____
_____
_____
_____
_____
_____

What is unique about me:

_____
_____
_____
_____
_____

What I love about my body.

How to Break a Fast

Greater than 24 hours

4-Step Process

1
BONE BROTH
Contains glycine that repairs the inner lining of the gut

2
PROBIOTIC FOOD
Replenishes the gut with good bacteria (sauerkraut, kombucha, yogurt, kimchi)

3
STEAMED VEGGIES
Provides fiber to the good bacteria

4
PROTEIN
Ready now for animal or plant protein

Note: You can plan for about 30 minutes between each step.

How to Break a
Shorter Fast to . . .

 Kill Hunger and Extend Fast

Break with **GOOD FAT**
- MCT oil
- grass-fed ghee or butter
- avocados
- nut butter
- fat bomb/keto cup
- Andreas seed oils

 Build More Muscle

Break with **PROTEIN**
- protein only (eggs, meat)

Note: A shorter fast is considered 24 hours or less.

 Keep Energy High

Break with **LIQUIDS**
- Organifi green or red juices
- Bone broth

 Heal Your Gut

Break with **PROBIOTICS**
- sauerkraut, kimchi, yogurt

BONUS GIFT

Let Dr. Mindy take you on an incredible journey in "A Love Letter from Your Body," a guided practice to enhance your fasting experience.

To access this bonus content, please visit www.hayhouse.com/download and enter the Product ID and Download Code as they appear below.

Product ID: 7870

Download Code: audio

For further assistance, please contact
Hay House Customer Care by phone:

US (800) 654-5126 or INTL CC+(760) 431-7695

or visit www.hayhouse.com/contact.

Thank you again for your Hay House purchase. Enjoy!

Hay House LLC • P.O. Box 5100

Carlsbad, CA 92018 • (800) 654-5126

• • •

Acknowledgments

My first thank you goes to YOU! After spending decades in the health trenches with thousands of women, listening to the health challenges so many of us go through, I decided it was time for me to take on the daunting task of writing a book that would change women's health forever. When I wrote *Fast Like a Girl*, the world was just emerging out of a pandemic that left so many of us grappling with fear, confusion, and a disbelief of our own healing power. As many of you have experienced, fasting is a free health tool that can be used by practically everyone and is so ridiculously effective that it also allows you to witness firsthand just how powerful your body is built to be.

Your enthusiasm has helped to get *Fast Like a Girl* into the hands of hundreds of thousands of women. Never in my wildest dreams did I think it would have that kind of impact so quickly. Not only did you pour onto my socials, but you have left amazing online reviews and shared the book with so many of your friends. Thank you for that! Together, we started a health movement for women. A movement that is allowing women to take their power back when it comes to their health. Please know that your commitment to learning all the miracles your hormonally driven body can perform has moved me deeply.

You are the reason I wrote this journal. I wanted to give you more tools to help you deepen your relationship with the inner intelligence that lives within every cell of your body. Your body has so much to tell you if you are willing to listen. Thank you for showing up for yourself, for your willingness to do the work, and for your compassion and willingness to share your discoveries with other women. We are definitely more powerful together!

I also have to give a huge thank you to my sweet friend and fellow author Alex Elle. When we met for the first time in person, a month after *Fast Like a Girl* was released, Alex encouraged me to write a journal that could be used while fasting. Alex's books are all aimed at helping us navigate our own emotional healing journeys. She is the master of teaching how to go within and shed light on the scary emotional places that live inside us. When this journal became a reality, Alex was my first choice for assistance in crafting the most impactful journal possible. Thank you, Alex, for your insight, collaboration on this project, and for caring so deeply about the healing process for us all. I adore you and loved working on this journal with you!

To my wise literary agent, Stephanie Tade, I am so grateful for your belief in me and for recognizing my mission to help women heal. You continue to

●●●

be a beautiful anchor of support for me as *Fast Like a Girl* has taken over the world. Thank you for always being willing to hop on a call, navigate the new territories I find myself in, and most of all for being a calming energy in what often feels like turbulent waters.

Lastly, to my Hay House family: Wow! Your support has meant the world to me! Thank ALL of you for not only helping me successfully launch *Fast Like a Girl* into the world but for seeing that other tools (like this journal) will deepen a woman's healing experience. Ever since I was a teenager, I've been reading Hay House books. The teachings in those books created the person I am today. I am BEYOND grateful to have found a publishing home with you. Can't wait to see what we dream up next!

● ● ●

About the Author

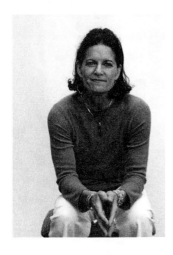

Dr. Mindy H. Pelz, DC, is the internationally best-selling author of *Fast Like a Girl* and *The Menopause Reset*. She is a nutrition and functional health expert who has spent more than two decades helping thousands of people successfully reclaim their health. She is a recognized leader in the alternative health field and a pioneer in the fasting movement, teaching the principles of a fasting lifestyle, diet variation, detox, hormones, and more. Her popular YouTube channel, where she regularly updates followers on the latest science-backed tools and techniques to help them reset their health, has 60 million lifetime views. She is the host of one of the leading science podcasts, *The Resetter Podcast*, has appeared on national shows like Extra TV and The Doctors, and has been featured in *Muscle & Fitness, Well + Good, SheKnows, Healthline*, and more.

To learn more about Dr. Mindy and her work, visit **drmindypelz.com**.

● ● ●

THE INTERNATIONAL BESTSELLING SENSATION

THAT LAUNCHED A

FASTING REVOLUTION!

BY LEADING NUTRITION AND FUNCTIONAL
HEALTH EXPERT, **DR. MINDY PELZ**

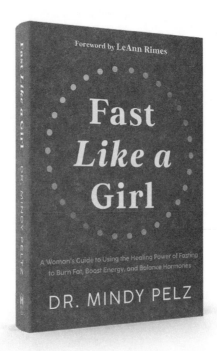

"At a time when all of us are looking for ways to improve
our health and vitality, Dr. Mindy Pelz offers great advice.
This book is about fasting, but also so much more. It's
about our womanhood, our health and our lives."

— **MARIANNE WILLIAMSON**, four-time
New York Times bestselling author

EXPERIENCE COMMUNITY AND COACHING WITH DR. MINDY'S RESET ACADEMY

The Reset Academy is for women who want help and support to successfully live a fasting lifestyle . . .

As well as home to a buzzing community of incredible women . . .

Where experienced coaches answer your burning questions about fasting, weight loss, or nutrition . . .

So you get the essential support to ensure embarking on the fasting lifestyle is a smooth and safe process.

To learn more about the Reset Academy visit:
resetacademy.drmindypelz.com

We hope you enjoyed this Hay House book. If you'd like to receive our online catalog featuring additional information on Hay House books and products, or if you'd like to find out more about the Hay Foundation, please contact:

Hay House LLC, P.O. Box 5100, Carlsbad, CA 92018-5100
(760) 431-7695 or (800) 654-5126
(760) 431-6948 (fax) or (800) 650-5115 (fax)
www.hayhouse.com® • www.hayfoundation.org

———

Published in Australia by: Hay House Australia Pty. Ltd.,
18/36 Ralph St., Alexandria NSW 2015
Phone: 612-9669-4299 • *Fax:* 612-9669-4144
www.hayhouse.com.au

Published in the United Kingdom by: Hay House UK, Ltd.,
The Sixth Floor, Watson House, 54 Baker Street, London W1U 7BU
Phone: +44 (0)20 3927 7290 • *Fax:* +44 (0)20 3927 7291
www.hayhouse.co.uk

Published in India by: Hay House Publishers India,
Muskaan Complex, Plot No. 3, B-2, Vasant Kunj, New Delhi 110 070
Phone: 91-11-4176-1620 • *Fax:* 91-11-4176-1630
www.hayhouse.co.in

———

Access New Knowledge.
Anytime. Anywhere.

Learn and evolve at your own pace
with the world's leading experts.

www.hayhouseU.com

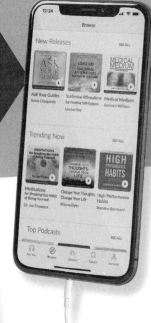